CORPORATE
SPINE

CORPORATE
SPINE

HOW SPINE SURGERY WENT OFF TRACK
AND HOW WE PUT IT RIGHT

ARDAVAN ASLIE, MD

Book layout by Reider Books
Cover design by Bigpoints

Publisher's Cataloging-in-Publication Data
provided by Five Rainbows Cataloging Services

Names: Aslie, Ardavan, author.
Title: Corporate spine : how spine surgery went off track and how we put it right / Ardavan Aslie.
Description: Sacramento, CA : SpineTall Press, 2022. | Includes bibliographical references and index.
Identifiers: LCCN 2022913041 (print) | ISBN 979-8-9864833-0-6 (paperback) | ISBN 979-8-9864833-1-3 (ebook)
Subjects: LCSH: Spine—Surgery. | Spinal fusion. | Back—Surgery. | Backache—Surgery. | Backache—Treatment. | BISAC: MEDICAL / Surgery / General.
Classification: LCC RD768 .A85 2022 (print) | LCC RD768 (ebook) | DDC 617.5/6059—dc23.

SpineTall Press
1111 Exposition Boulevard
Building 500B
Sacramento, CA 95815

Printed in the United States of America

To my wife, my mother, my sister, my three daughters, and to equal rights and equal pay for every woman in this world, no matter their country, no matter their religion, and no matter their culture.

Table of Contents

Acknowledgements

I would like to thank my lovely wife, who put up with me for the better part of two years when my mind was constantly occupied with this book project.

I would also like to thank my orthopedic chairman, who told me that I'm a dreamer, and that it's always the dreamers who come up with inventions—not the guys who win awards. He told me to keep dreaming big.

Thank you also, JP, for your inspiration and help in writing this book.

Special Acknowledgements

I would like to take a moment to thank the dedicated men and women who have served in our Armed Forces. I would also like to thank the first responders who protect us, including firefighters, law enforcement, and EMTs. Without them, my life would be considerably worse, and I owe them all an enormous debt of gratitude.

For most of my life, I was willing to sacrifice a good life for hard work. When I was in Berkeley, I went through quite an ordeal to make sure I finished my junior and senior years with a double major. In medical school, while my classmates were having a good time, I was doing nothing but studying. In my life, I have looked up to many of my professors and successful people outside my specialty, people like Jeff Bezos or Tom Brady, but I have never envied anyone except one—his name was Michael Monsoor, a US Navy Seal and Medal of Honor recipient. Michael saved two of his comrades by jumping on a grenade. He did not make that selfless decision right when he saw the grenade; he had already made that decision years earlier when he was a young man. People like Michael Monsoor may no longer be with us, but they do not die. They become part of all of us and live forever. I envy him because he got a chance to show his bravery at a level that people might not even understand. Only a person who has decided that they will live for other people can know such a mindset.

Disclaimer

This book contains the opinions and ideas of its author. It is intended to provide helpful and informative material on the subject addressed in the book. It is sold with the understanding that the author is not engaged in rendering medical, health, or any other kind of personal professional services in the book. The reader should consult with his or her medical, health, or other competent professional before adopting any of the suggestions in this book or drawing inferences from it. The author specifically disclaims all responsibility for any liability, loss, or risk, personal or otherwise, which is incurred as a consequence, directly or indirectly, of the use and application of any of the contents of this book.

Introduction

December 29, 2020—My blood oxygen saturation dropped to 80 percent as I lay in an ICU bed suffering from a severe case of COVID-19. Despite all the oxygen blowing into my nose and face, my saturation number stubbornly refused to rise. Five doctors and nurses worked on me frantically, doing everything humanly possible to save my life. Because of my medical training, I knew precisely what was going on, what they were trying to do, and how close to death I really was. In utter panic and with labored breathing, I turned to one of my nurses and said, "Please do not let me die. I have to save spine surgery." Perhaps she thought I was delusional or delirious, but I was far from it. It was a moment of absolute and total clarity.

The philosopher Friedrich Nietzsche once famously said, "He who has a why to live for can bear almost any how." As my body began to shut down, I realized that the need to save spine surgery was my why. That very thought infused new life into me. Five days after nearly dying, I was discharged from the hospital. Two months of recovery later, I rewrote this entire manuscript.

In this book, I will explain how a simple comment led to an award-winning invention. That development led me to revisit the entire biomechanics of spine surgery, which in turn pushed me to ask hard questions about my subspecialty. The search for answers and truth guided me to uncover what I believe is a deep conspiracy in orthopedic surgery. I decided that the best way to convey this information to my audience would be through a simplified primer on spine surgery. Chapters One through Four are meant to teach the general public about the basics of spine surgery and the difficulties surgeons encounter. I hope that readers will use this information to ask better questions and understand the pros and cons of different procedures.

In Chapters Five, Seven, and Eight, I discuss how medical device companies have successfully taken over the specialty of spine surgery and driven it into a dead end. This is a dead end where pockets get filled and patients get no benefit. At the center of this discussion are large screws (pedicle screws) that are being used as bone anchors.

In Chapter Six, I digress momentarily to explain my personal story and how this journey unraveled. I went from student to practitioner to researcher to bio-mechanic to inventor and eventually to warrior.

Even though this book is directed toward people with no medical training, I felt it necessary to write down the specific biomechanics of spine surgery, just in case—and perhaps in hopes that—another spine surgeon will read this book. (I invite lay readers who wish to learn more to visit my website, www.corporatespinebook.com. It includes videos that complement each chapter and go into further detail on key topics and ideas addressed in the book.)

For years, I tried every avenue possible to get the message out to my fellow physicians, but my words fell on deaf ears. Writing this book, even if no one reads it, will at least clear my conscience. I have stood up for the truth and have done everything within my power to warn people. Without course correction, there will be no progress in spine surgery, and I promise we will be doing the exact same surgeries decades from now, with no clear improvement in patient outcomes.

Unraveling the apparent conspiracy of medical device companies, as huge as it was, was only the tip of the iceberg. I came to understand that the real problems are our lack of core understanding of biomechanics and of the practice of spine surgery. As a subspecialty of orthopedic surgery, we used our knowledge and methods for the treatment of long bone fractures and applied them to spinal fusions. When our studies came back and said this was wrong, we looked the other way, especially when it came to the culture that instrument companies created.

However, there is good news. Over the last five years, I have discovered and written about biomechanics that are specific to the spine. Now we also have the necessary tools that will enable us to make appropriate devices for spinal bone anchors. With laser drilling, 3D printing, and advancements in material technology, we can build devices that were not possible even just a decade ago.

Before we can do anything else, however, we must loosen the grip that medical device companies have on the science of spine surgery. The so-called consultants need to understand that no matter how much they believe in a certain technology, they must be impartial and evaluate every device without bias. In addition, they must stop writing favorably biased papers for medical device companies. Only then can spine surgery get back on track to being an efficient and life-changing specialty of medicine.

CHAPTER ONE

Anatomy of the Spine

To get the most out of the discussion in this book, I want you to understand the spine. My descriptions may seem technical, but I will be discussing basic anatomy and will explain the subject just as I would if you came to me as a patient. My goal is to make you a more educated consumer of medical goods and services. The more you know, the better your chances of getting informed and optimal medical care.

The spine connects the skull to the pelvis and has three regions. First is the cervical spine, which has seven vertebrae, known as C1–C7. In the middle, there is the thoracic spine, which has twelve vertebrae, T1–T12. The lumbar spine has five vertebrae, L1–L5. The lumbar spine attaches to the sacrum, a single bone that is part of both the pelvis and the spine. The sacrum connects on top to the fifth lumbar vertebra through the disc in the middle, and it also connects on both sides to the ilium, which are the hip bones that you feel on your sides.

Before I go further into the anatomy of the spine, I need to explain a little bit of its function. Different areas of the spine have different

Anatomy of the Vertebral Column

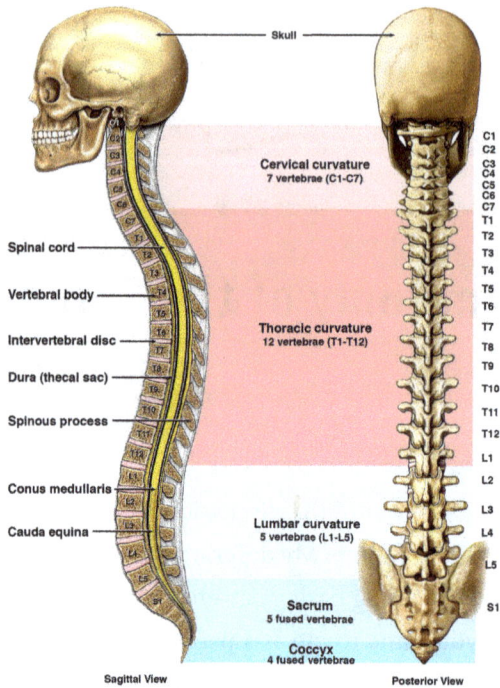

Figure 1: Anatomy of the Vertebral Column (Spine)

functions. Their motion is specialized to perform that function, which also affects their shape.

For example, the thoracic spine aids in respiration, supports the ribcage, and houses vital organs. The cervical spine supports the head's range of motion and position The lumbar spine supports the trunk and transmits the force of gravity into the pelvis.

Range of motion is important in the lumbar spine but not as important as it is in the cervical spine. The thoracic spine is relatively immobile because of attachment to the rib cage. However, the mobility of the thoracolumbar junction—where the thoracic and lumbar spine meet—makes it more vulnerable to injury. The range of motion of the lumbar spine is limited compared to the cervical spine. Most people think that bending forward to touch their hands to the ground is lumbar flexion. In fact, most of that flexion comes from the hip joints. I have patients that have multiple levels fused in the lumbar spine but still can bend and touch the ground. Stability is much more important in the lumbar spine than range of motion. This is an extremely important point, which we will review in detail later.

The spine has two important functions. One is structural support. We are upright mammals; we walk only on our feet and use our hands to perform tasks. The spine must support the entire body. The second function of the spine is to protect neural structures. These are the pathways that connect the brain to the rest of the body, including the upper and lower extremities, via the spinal cord.

The spinal cord is not just a cable that connects the brain to the rest of the body; it is a computer. When you perform repetitious tasks, like tapping your foot or walking, the movements that we do unconsciously are all coordinated by reflexes in the spinal cord, which does not tolerate compression very much. However, the peripheral nerves that come out of the spinal cord and go to the extremities are just cables that connect the central nervous system to the rest of the body. They tolerate compression a lot more than the spinal cord.

The spinal cord comes from the brain, goes through the spinal canal, and ends right around the L1–L2 area. From that point, the nerves come down to form what we call *cauda equina*, a horse's tail. Therefore, from L2 down to S1, the spinal cord does not exist. Only the nerves, which look like a bunch of spaghetti, come down from the spinal cord and through the spinal canal. This is important because some of the injections in that area from L2 down are very safe, and there is little danger of damaging the spinal cord.

Let's focus for a moment on the cervical spine, which has seven vertebrae. The first two vertebrae, C1 and C2, have an unusual and very specialized anatomy that is beyond the scope of this book to detail. From

Vertebral body

Superior
articular
process

Transverse
process

Spinous process

Vertebral
foramen

Pedicle

Lamina

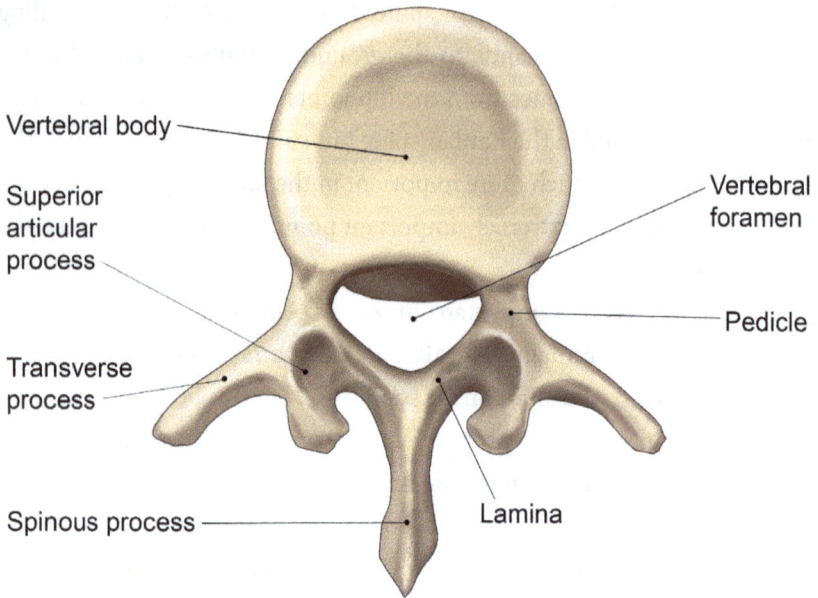

Figure 2: Lumbar Vertebra

C3 down to C7, the cervical spinal vertebrae look more like you might expect a vertebra to look.

The cervical spine has a third function that the thoracic and lumbar spine do not have: allowing the head to move. Fifty percent of the range of motion of the head comes from where the skull meets the cervical spine. Therefore, if we fused the entire cervical spine, the patient would still retain 50 percent of the overall range of motion of the head.

The typical spinal vertebra has two segments. One is a block of bone that is meant to carry weight, called the vertebralbody. The outside shell is dense, strong cortical bone, and the inside is spongy bone. The vertebral body size increases as we go from the top of the spine to the bottom of the spine because the lower region must carry more weight. Two cylinder-like columns project backward from each vertebra. The outside of these projections is dense cortical bone, and the inside bone is again spongy bone. We call these columns *pedicles*.

The forces from the muscles that manipulate and move the spine get transferred from the attachments at the back of the vertebra into the pedicle and then into the vertebral body. Therefore, the pedicle is a structure of force transfer. The pedicles connect to each other with two flat bones that form a shape almost like the top of an archway into a garden, and we call these *lamina*. There is one on each side of the vertebra, and they connect to each other in the middle.

A lamina is one of the strongest bones in the body, and pretty much all of it is dense cortical bone. To continue my analogy, the columns that hold up the archway are the pedicles. The top of the archway that connects at an angle is the lamina. The vertebral body is the stone that you step on to pass through the gate. When you stack vertebrae on top of each other, these archways line up to form a canal that extends from the top of the cervical spine, near the brain, all the way to the sacrum. This canal protects the spinal cord from outside forces.

As the spinal cord travels down from the brain to the middle of the spinal canal, nerves branch off of the spinal cord and go under the pedicle at each level between two vertebrae. The nerves then go out toward the upper extremity or lower extremity where they have to innervate.

The opening between one pedicle and the next lower-level pedicle is called *neural foramina*. This is basically a "nerve hole," if I were to translate. At each level, there are neural foramina that nerves from the spinal cord pass through. That means that if the disc (which we will explain in the next section) gets injured and there is loss of height between the vertebrae, the two pedicles get closer to each other, and the nerve that is coming out between them can be pinched. That is where the term "pinched nerve" comes from. Of course, a nerve can be pinched by a herniated disc as well.

There are three protrusions that extend outward like an antenna from the back of the vertebra: one on each side, and one is straight back. The one straight back is called the *spinous process*, and the ones on each side are called *transverse processes*. These are attachment points for the paraspinal muscles, and their function is to allow the muscles to move the spine in three-dimensional space according to what the person would like to do. These processes do not have very good quality bone, and they are not very important in terms of surgical treatments.

Each vertebra in the spine connects to the vertebra above and vertebra below at three points. This is probably because, in nature, three points of contact is the most efficient way to stabilize a structure.

By convention, the spinal canal is the dividing section of the spinal structure. Anything in front of the spinal canal is called the front, and anything behind it is called the back. In the front, one vertebra connects to the vertebrae through the discs above and below. The footprint of the disc, which we will discuss below, is very similar to the footprint and shape of the vertebral body in its cross-section. Therefore, the disc does not protrude beyond the bone border.

Discs

The next structure I would like to talk about is the cushion between each vertebra, which we call a *disc*. This is the most important structure in the world of spine surgery, as this is the structure most damaged by wear and tear or mechanical injury, which causes pain. From cervical vertebra number two, or C2, all the way down to the sacrum, every vertebra is separated from the one below or above by one of these discs. The disc has a very complex structure and very complex innervation. To be truthful, we do not understand this structure very well. Just when you think you have a grip and are starting to understand, you realize you have entered a new room with many unknowns. The invention of the MRI in 1980 was significant for the world of spine surgery. It was the MRI that enabled us to see the discs and therefore diagnose problems.

Each disc is normally composed of two structures. One is the gelatinous material in the middle that is very soft and mushy, called the *nucleus pulposus*. The second structure is a tough ring that surrounds the nucleus pulposus and supports the gelatinous material. Together, they functions as a shock absorber.

The disc has two equally important functions. One is motion. Because these discs are flexible, it allows two vertebrae to move against each other, and therefore the spine can move in three dimensions. The second function is stability. When the disc is healthy, it holds the two bones together, separated from each other but snug against the disc. However, when the disc is damaged, the two vertebrae slip and settle on each other, causing all sorts of impingement of the nerves and potentially pain.

The disc is highly innervated, and its integrity is very important. I would say it is almost like a tire. When the tire is intact, it can hold the pressure of the air inside it very well. In discs, instead of air, we have the gelatinous material in the middle. However, if the disc gets subjected to forces that exceed its capability or threshold, then the strong *annulus fibrosus*—the tough exterior of the disc—can tear.

A lot of things can happen when the disc sustains an injury, and what exactly happens has a lot to do with the size of the tear. If the disc is injured by a very large force and has a very large tear, the gelatinous material in the middle of the disc can get blown out, just like a tire with a large puncture. But a lot of times, the tear is very small and sometimes even undetectable with an MRI. I tell my patients this is like a small nail in a tire. On many occasions, I have checked my tire for few days and cannot tell if it is deflating. By the third or fourth day, I realize the tire has been deflating, and it has settled, and it turns out there was a small nail in the tire. If that is the case in the spine, it takes months to years for the disc to deflate and start settling.

I am not going to get into specifics. One of the reasons I say this is that, truthfully, we do not understand the specifics. Overall, we know that there are two ways that an injured disc can cause pain. However, we do not understand the pain pathways very well. We do know that when the disc sustains an injury, the disc itself becomes painful. This is what we call *discogenic pain*. This pain shows itself mostly as what we call *axial pain*, which is basically the pain in the center of the spine: either the neck, thoracic, mid-back, or lower back pain. This pain can travel down the legs or the arms. But the pain is primarily in the back.

The second way a disc can cause pain is by irritating the nerves around it. In this situation, the material inside the disc escapes and gets ejected into the canal, where it is not supposed to be. This is what we call *disc herniation* or *bulge*. This creates two problems. One is the actual compression or pinching of the nerves. In this situation, the electrical transmission through the nerve gets interrupted, and the patient feels numbness and weakness in the distribution of that specific nerve. The second thing that can happen when a disc contacts a nerve is that the material inside the disc is an irritant to the nerves. When the nerve gets irritated, then the patient feels pain in the distribution of that nerve in the form of stabbing or burning pain in the extremity. It is generally referred to as *sciatica* in the lower extremity.

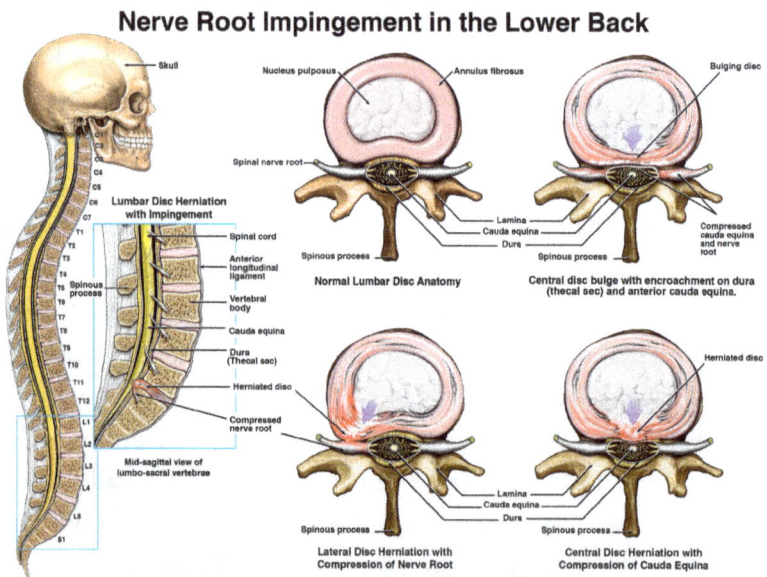

**Figure 3: Classic Lumbar Disc Herniation
with Nerve Root Impingement**

Overall, we do not understand the cascade of events that ends up in pain perception. We do know that it has something to do with inflammation. I always tell my patients that the goal is to reduce inflammation. The way I explain it is that most of the time in chronic conditions, it is not the damage that causes the pain; it is the body's attempt to repair the damage—which is inflammation—that causes it.

Normally inflammation has a very bad connotation. When something is inflamed, we want to do what we can to decrease or eliminate the inflammation. In actuality, inflammation is the body's repair mechanism, or the body's construction site. Pain in itself is not bad. The analogy I use is that when you try to build an apartment building, the first thing you do is place a fence around the construction site so that people can do their jobs. I say that the pain is something similar. Pain lets a person decrease their activities so the repair mechanisms can do their job. If there is no pain and a person continues with full activity, this aggravates the area and does not allow for repair.

This is a very big and controversial topic in the world of medicine in terms of what to do with inflammation. Some doctors say that we should not reduce inflammation because it is the repair mechanism. My perception of inflammation in the spine is that, unfortunately, the body does not have an effective mechanism to repair the discs because it cannot fight gravity. The body tries and tries, but it is not successful.

One of the common questions patients ask me is if this disc will heal itself and get better with some therapy. I tell them no. The only way to fix it is either to travel to outer space and be weightless in a laboratory at a space station or to suspend yourself in the air for months at a time. When the inflammation and the repair mechanisms do not have the power to repair the problem, then the repair mechanism becomes the main problem itself. In this situation, we are trying to tell the body to stop trying. That is why anti-inflammatory injections are one of the most powerful tools we have for the treatment of neck and back pain.

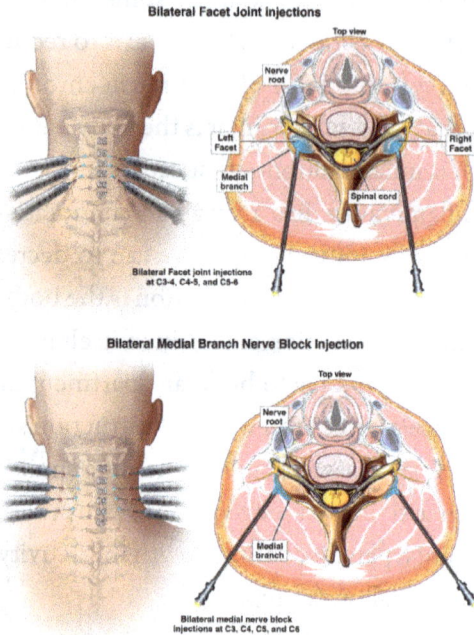

Figure 4: Cervical Spine Injections

How does the disc get injured? Of course, every disc in every person has a certain appearance. As we discussed, the fibrotic ring that holds the gelatinous nucleus together is made of collagen fibers. If the disc is subjected to forces that exceed its capacity, that is when it fails or tears. This could be due to any force in different directions from different types of accidents. It could be falling off a horse. It could be a motor vehicle accident. When the body gets thrown forward or backward, meaning it gets loaded axially, the stress goes right through the disc. Depending on the magnitude of this destructive force and the direction it comes from, the disc can tear. The disc can technically tear on the front side or the back; however, it is the tear at the back, which is close to the nerves, that becomes the most symptomatic.

This is where things get very complicated. The disc has two aspects that affect its strength. One is the anatomical and structural appearance. Basically, every person's discs are different in height and thickness. That is something that you can see on MRIs. I have patients that have very thin discs and patients that have very thick discs. The other aspect is at the molecular level. You cannot see the molecular crosslinking of the collagen on an MRI. Some of the collagen is very strong and heavily crosslinked, and some collagen is weak without significant crosslinking. That means even though two discs can look very similar in different people, the infrastructure can be very different with different strengths. That is what makes everyone different. Just as nobody's face is exactly the same, that is also how the back is.

Because the spine has different curvatures and gets loaded in different manner, each level of the disc has a very different strength that is specific for that location along the length of the spine. Therefore, it is almost impossible to come up with a number for how much force it would take for a disc to get disrupted. Even if you hypothetically determine that number for a certain disc, I can tell you that the number that leads to the failure of that disc is specific to that disc only and does not even apply to the disc above or below it, let alone to the same disc in somebody else.

I occasionally have to testify for my patients in lawsuits, where I will hear a bioengineer state that he has calculated the forces applied to my patient's body and my patient could not have been injured. These statements are so wrong, for many reasons. It is impossible to calculate the force that injures each disc in each person simply because we do not know the molecular structure of each disc.

These attributes are what make spine surgery unique in medicine. The spine is both frustrating and beautiful. It is frustrating because it is very difficult to come up with a standardized treatment for everyone. It is beautiful because our job is not boring at all—far from it. Throughout our careers, we develop skills as spine surgeons that can direct treatment to different patients in an individualized fashion. During the first ten years of my practice, just about everyone received cookie-cutter treatment. But as I advanced in my career, I learned to apply specific treatment courses to a specific person with a specific problem. That takes decades to learn.

I can tell you that the disc is a very complex structure in terms of supporting the spine and the weight of the body, and the disc is inherently a stable structure. That is a very important concept that is very hard for many surgeons to understand.

Facet Joints

Each vertebra connects to the vertebra above and below through facet joints. Every vertebra has two bony processes that extend up and then two bony processes that extend down. The bony process that extends up articulates with the two bony processes that come down from the vertebra above, and these form a facet joint.

These facet joints are just like any other joint in the body in that they are lined with what is called *hyaline cartilage*. They are the size of the knuckles in your hands, and one is present on each side of the vertebra. The orientation and shape of the facet joints dictate how one vertebra moves relative to the vertebra above and vertebra below.

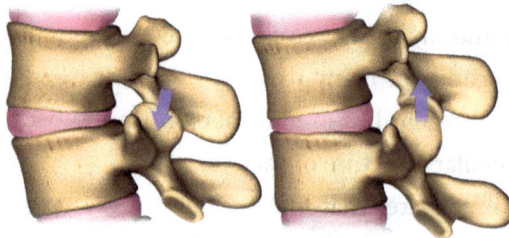

Figure 5: Side View of Working Facet Joints

In the cervical spine, where we want the widest range of motion, these facet joints are relatively horizontally oriented. This orientation gives more freedom to the disc and enables it to move one vertebra in relation to another. This increases the range of motion of the cervical spine.

In the lumbar spine, the facet joints become almost vertical. This orientation makes the lumbar spine stable and does not allow a significant range of motion. The motion of one vertebra relative to another vertebra in this lower part of the spine is rotational. If there is any translation, meaning one vertebra slips forward and back over another vertebra, we call that a *pathological condition* and, therefore, *instability*.

Just like any other structure that moves in the body, these facet joints can break down. I will talk about the conditions of the spine in the next section. For now, I just need you to understand that the orientation of the facet joints dictates what type of motion you get from one vertebra relative to the vertebra next to it.

Orientation of the Spine

The cervical spine has seven vertebrae, and as I noted, the first two have a unique appearance while the remaining five resemble each other. The thoracic spine has twelve vertebrae that look very similar to each other, but they are different as you go from top to bottom. The lumbar spine has five vertebrae, and they are similar-looking overall. The sacrum at the bottom is one large bone. The sacrum connects to the ilium on the sides to form the pelvis.

Each region has a particular curve that is special to it. If you look at somebody from the side, you can see that the cervical spine curves backward. This is called *cervical lordosis*. The thoracic spine curves forward, which is called *thoracic kyphosis*. The lumbar spine curves backward again, and this is called *lumbar lordosis*.

Why do we have these curvatures? In a four-legged mammal, the structure of the spine is much simpler. For them, the spine runs along the back of the body, and the organs hang down from it. However, humans are upright mammals, and that makes things significantly more complicated.

The entire goal of human evolution is to have the most efficient and balanced spinal structure so the muscles will work the least when we stand upright. If the organs were all on one side of the spine, we would need very large muscles on the other side. To accommodate organs like the lungs, heart, and abdominal contents, the spine must fall into a specific curvature.

The thoracic spine is the most responsible for this. It holds the ribcage, which allows the lungs to move in a rhythmic motion for respiration. This part of the spine must be kyphotic, or curving forward. With this part of the spine curving forward, the rest of the spine needs to compensate for that. That is why we have cervical and lumbar lordosis.

The whole goal is that the spine must be balanced so that the center of gravity falls either on or extremely close to the base of the spine. This way, the muscles work the least amount to hold a person upright. This concept is very important to understand, because when we do treatments of the spine surgically, we must make sure that if the body has gone out of alignment, it will be restored. If you are performing surgery on the spine, this alignment must be maintained. That is what we learn when we go through our training and fellowship.

Throughout life, humans go through different stages. At some stages we are active, and as we enter middle age and later life, our activities decrease and we become more sedentary. Of course, it is very difficult to maintain the spine throughout all decades of life, but it is important to discuss it.

Weight is very important in terms of spine function. More weight means more stress on the spine and discs. In my twenty years of practice, I have not found a way of discussing weight that does not upset patients. Most of the time, the patient is very aware of the problem, and they have tried weight-loss remedies in the past that have not worked for them. For me to talk about this topic is also a difficult issue. Lots of people consider excess weight to have a behavioral component, but to a large extent I consider weight issues to be metabolic. Everyone knows that if you eat too much, you will probably gain weight. But it's not that simple. Your appetite and how much you eat is controlled by a center in the brain called the hypothalamus. Therefore, the urge to eat is but one component in a metabolic cascade that starts in the hypothalamus. Unfortunately, not everyone is born with a good metabolism.

We need to talk about the mechanics of excess weight. When somebody is overweight, they can have adipose tissue, or fat tissue, in the buttocks, thighs, or other areas of the body, but this commonly appears in the abdominal area. To compensate for this excess weight, the back muscles must work harder to keep the back straight. Because these muscles are closer to the spine, they must work a lot harder. The excess abdominal weight is in the belly, so it is far away from the spine.

Think of the spine in this case as a flagpole. For a flagpole to stay upright, the pull from different cables have to cancel each other out. Your back muscles and abdominal weight are like those cables attached to the flagpole. When it comes to extra weight in the belly, the more force that is created, the more the back muscles have to pull to counterbalance that force. If you have one pound of excess weight in your gut, the back muscles must pull down on the spine to try to balance it with two to three pounds of force, due to the weight's distance from the spine. Losing one or two pounds from the gut means taking two to four pounds off the spine. This is simple physics: both the muscles and extra weight pull down on the spine, so they add on to each other. This makes heavier patients more susceptible to injury.

Imagine a person is involved in a car accident. In this situation, the head and trunk get thrown back and forth violently, and all this stress gets dissipated right through the discs in the base of the spine. In heavier patients, therefore, the discs are more prone to injury. It is also much more difficult for a heavy patient to recover because multiple factors may slow their recovery. They are sometimes stuck in a no-win situation.

Prevention is the best option, of course, and there are many ways to maintain good bone quality as we age. Eating healthy is very important. We also need to have routine exercise, mostly in the form of cardio exercise. That allows for better oxygenation in the blood and better-toned muscles.

Muscle balance is very important for spine health. We do know that the spine can get out of alignment very quickly in people with muscle issues, and some patients develop a significant curvature that can impede vital activities, such as breathing.

My guidelines are that patients should regularly do an activity that they enjoy and that they can continue into advanced age. In addition, it should not be exercise that puts pressure on the back. The exercises that I like at the gym are pullups, pulldowns, stationary biking, and low-impact exercises, such as the Stairmaster or elliptical machines. When it comes to weightlifting, my recommendation is to use less weight and more repetition. I have been taught by my trainer that you can do a great workout and burn a lot of calories with just two to three pounds. You do not have to lift fifteen to twenty pounds to get good exercise. Lifting heavy weight causes damage to the joints.

I have patients who are not professional athletes but want to do a heavy amount of exercise. I tell them that they could end up paying for this activity later in life. Now that I am fifty-five years old, my perspective of life has completely changed. I always tell my patients that in my twenties, I wanted to look big, and now in my fifties, I just want to look small. Unfortunately, I have carried some of the injuries that I received in my twenties, and to this day, this occasionally causes problems for me. I tell my young patients in their late teens or early twenties that the goal should be to keep their body healthy enough to enjoy their retirement years.

Bone quality is important for two reasons. One reason is that it is possible that the vertebral body—which looks like a square from the side, or like a cylinder—starts settling. Instead of a square, it starts to look like a wedge. This is probably due to microfractures that occur throughout the lifespan with daily activities. Over time, the thoracic spine could start settling into a more kyphotic, or forward-curving, form. To compensate, the cervical spine and the lumbar spine start to settle more into lordosis, or backward-curving, form. Once this cascade happens, it is almost like a runaway train that is very difficult to stop. The process happens over decades, and it happens to people that have poor-quality bone to begin with; therefore, the treatment options are very limited.

The other problem that can happen is what we call compression fracture. At some point in life, the bone gets so weak that it cannot stand even moderate activities performed by an individual. In that situation, the vertebral body gets crushed. I have seen many patients that end up getting multiple compression fractures with advanced age. This starts the same cascade of changing spinal curvature over again, except a lot worse, and treatment of this condition is very difficult.

Compression fractures are what pushed me to start my research and development into new surgical devices. I knew that with the population aging, this sort of weak bone quality among older people posed a significant health morbidity threat. The current devices we have in terms of metal screws are just a no-win situation. When a bone gets that weak, the screw slices through it like a hot knife going through butter. My goal was to invent a device that will have a chance of correcting and fixing the issue in this population. That was my only intention when I started my research and development. However, that research and development led to another finding, and another finding, and another finding. As it progressed, the issue got bigger and bigger. I eventually uncovered a massive problem that we have faced all along. I will be explaining this topic in detail in the upcoming chapters.

Trying to find a way of maintaining bone quality in the elderly is a very active area of research in the world of medicine. We have come up with different medications and supplements over the years. Each one of these initially showed success, but eventually showed they did not make much difference.

As we wait for better treatments, I can say today that a good diet and routine exercise are absolutely essential to maintaining normal alignment of the spine.

Paraspinal Muscles

So far, we have talked about basic anatomy of the spine and have defined the anatomy of the vertebrae and how they connect to each other. We have talked about the overall alignment of the spine, the importance of it, and what we can do to maintain that alignment. Next, I will briefly touch on a very difficult topic that we do not know much about: paraspinal muscles.

In medical school, when I was studying anatomy, we studied the muscles in the extremities in depth, and I had detailed knowledge of them. I was anticipating this topic to become more difficult when we got to the paraspinal muscles. But it was the complete opposite. We pretty much did not study it. The paraspinal muscles were just ignored.

The paraspinal muscles are a combination of many very strong muscles acting in different directions, and they have a very complex structure. They just happen to be all in the back of the spine. They span from the skull all the way down to the pelvis. These muscles are responsible for the motion of the entire trunk. They have a very complex task, which is orienting the entire trunk in a three-dimensional space in a smooth manner. As a matter of fact, the only way we can differentiate them is by the fact that there are three layers of paraspinal muscles. Other than that, there is not much of a differentiation.

In addition, we do not have very good imaging to study these muscles. An MRI can only differentiate layers of muscle, and that is about it. It does not show the origin and attachments of these muscles individually. However, we know that the function of the paraspinal muscles is very important because, unfortunately, in children with muscular dystrophy or difficulty with muscle strength, imbalance and severe scoliosis

22

sets in at very early ages. Normally, these situations require massive surgical intervention with very large fusions so the patient can at least sit up.

One thing that we know very well is the amount of damage that is inflicted on the paraspinal muscles during open spinal surgeries. To perform a fusion at a certain level, we make a midline incision and just go down through the fascia. Once we get to the spinous processes, where the muscles attach to the bones, our next action as surgeons is to scrape the paraspinal muscles off the vertebra so we can perform our surgery. If pedicle screws are placed, we must scrape the muscle off the vertebra from edge to edge.

Sometimes we must dissect even further. When we must do quite a bit of work in the middle of the spine, there is nowhere to place your bone graft for the fusion but in the fusion gutters. The fusion gutters are an area that is beyond the facet joint, beyond the lamina, and between the transverse processes. This is a massive dissection with degloving of paraspinal muscles, which means basically detaching the muscles from the spine.

We know three things happen with this dissection. One, a good chunk of the muscle becomes denervated. We know very well that if you dissect the muscles beyond the facet joints, which we must do when we are putting pedicle screws in, it denervates the paraspinal muscle in that segment. Two, when we put our screws in, the screws impede the paraspinal muscles' reattachment to the bone. Even if there is an area that would allow them to reattach, the reattachment forms as scar tissue and not the strong tendons that they had before the surgery. Three, the surgery introduces a significant amount of scar tissue into the muscle itself. The combination of denervation detachment and scar tissue causes significant dysfunction of the paraspinal muscles. Each time you go back to do more dissection, more and more damage is inflicted on the paraspinal muscles.

I believe that once we do the dissection in surgery, three zones occur in the paraspinal muscles. The first zone is the immediate zone that has been scraped off the bone, and I believe this part of the muscle dies and turns into scar tissue. There is also a middle zone of muscle that has survived the insult of the surgery. It is scarred to the point that circulation into the muscle is compromised, but the muscle has not died off. Of course, the third zone, which is the farthest away from the dissection, is alive and well.

I believe the outcome of each surgery has a lot to do with what happens in the middle zone. That is very different from patient to patient and even side to side in the same patient. In the dead zone, when the muscle dies and turns into scar tissue, I do not believe that causes any problem. I do not believe the healthy zone, or outside zone, is a problem either. However, I believe we have significant issues with the zone in between, which I call the *transitional zone*.

In the transitional zone, the muscles are alive, but due to scar tissue, the blood supply is compromised. This is where the constant "charley horse" feeling comes from—the achy pain patients have after spinal surgery. Of course, the size of the zone dictates the amount of pain after surgical intervention. If this zone is small, between the dead zone and the live zone, then the patient does well. However, if this zone is larger, these are the patients that end up with postoperative pain that is different from their preoperative pain.

Of course, the big question is why we do these surgeries. If the surgery is going to exchange one pain for another pain, how can this field even exist? That can easily be explained by the nature and intensity of pain. Normally, the indication for spinal surgery is a pinched nerve or an injured disc. In these situations, the pain is sharp and sometimes unbearable. The pain becomes constant, and worst of all, does not respond to pain medication.

Sometimes I tell my patients that once they have a pinched nerve, they can take all the narcotics until they are barely breathing, but they are still not going to relieve that pain. These are the reasons that drive a patient to request and proceed with spinal procedures. However, postoperative pain, which I believe sometimes—not always—comes from the transitional zone in the paraspinal muscles, is a dull, achy pain, which responds well to local treatments and pain medication. This is a much more manageable problem than the problem that existed before the surgery. That is what most of my patients describe to me. My patients say that they are very happy with the results of surgery and the stabbing pain is resolved; however, they do have some dull, achy pain over the surgical area.

This amount of trauma to the paraspinal muscles was one of the reasons that we started transitioning into minimally invasive surgeries, and this technology has helped my patients significantly. We can place screws or do the surgery through small incisions. Minimally invasive surgery is mostly applicable to the lumbar spine. This is still up for debate, but a significant amount of spine surgery is being done traditionally, with dissection of paraspinal muscles, from corner to corner, off the spine.

The issue of destroying viable muscle was another reason that I proceeded with my research and development. Placement of the screws requires extensive dissection, and I wanted to come up with a device that required much less dissection. I will be talking about this in much more detail in the upcoming chapters.

I would like you to understand for now that the paraspinal muscles are one of the key elements of spinal function, and we know very little about them. One of the ways that we can learn more about them would be the future invention of imaging studies that can study the paraspinal muscles in a better way. For now, the best practice is to perform the surgeries with the least amount of dissection and to use techniques that do not disturb the function of the paraspinal muscles.

~

CHAPTER TWO

Conditions of the Spine

C onditions of the spine are very connected to the anatomy of the spine. In the body, whatever moves can become injured and subsequently cause pain, which is true of the spine as well.

The invention of the MRI gave spine surgeons a great tool for diagnosing and subsequently treating a lot of back ailments. Before the MRI, we had only X-rays, which provided images only of dense bone. The CT (computer tomography) scan was first commercially available in 1972, and the first MRI machine was available in 1979. These two inventions were the turning point for the diagnosis and treatment of spinal conditions because they allowed doctors to see more. However, they differ significantly in terms of what information they give the surgeon.

With the CT scan, the patient lies in a tube. As the patient's body is moved automatically through the tube, an X-ray beam circles around the body. On the opposite side is a sensor that detects the X-ray that has passed through the body. Based on those measurements, the scanner is able to recreate sliced images of the body. However, because a CT scan uses X-rays, the information is only as good as what X-ray images can show us. A CT scan is good for showing the bone, so for example, if there is trauma, the CT scan is a great way to detect any fractures.

One of the first tests we do when a patient comes to the emergency room after an accident is a CT scan of the area where we suspect injury. The CT scan also gives images of the soft tissue, such as the nerves and the discs, but these images are of very limited use.

One of the problems with the CT scan is that the patient receives radiation. If the patient is very young, especially a young girl, this could be detrimental. The positive thing about a CT scan is that it is readily available in the United States, and it is quick. It only takes five to ten minutes to scan the whole body. As a surgeon, I mostly use CT scans to see the position of my hardware after surgery, and it's the first thing I order (besides more general X-rays) if there is a trauma patient in the emergency room.

The MRI is the key imaging study used in spine surgery. In the 1980s and '90s, there was a significant improvement in MRI quality. For an MRI, the patient goes inside a tight tube, and sometimes patients can become claustrophobic. The machine has a very large magnet that is on all the time, and the magnetism spins protons in the body out of alignment. When the protons spin back to their original positions, they give off a wavelength. This wavelength can be picked up by MRI sensors, which are looking for water. In this way, the machine can calculate the water content in any area of the body. The areas that have more water appear white on the images, and the areas with less water appear dark. Different tissues, such as bone, cartilage, and nerves, have different water content.

With the proper software, when the signals are reconstructed, the MRI machine can produce images of internal organs. These slices can be in different planes, in axial, sagittal, or coronal views. There are also different wavelengths of imaging, called T1 or T2, which look for different structures. In my practice, I can get the most information from T2 sagittal views. This is the image in which the patient's body plane is divided in half from right to left. In this image, the cerebrospinal fluid appears light. Sometimes I look at the other images as well if I have a question, but this is my favorite view when I evaluate patients.

The downside of an MRI is the cost. The machines are very expensive, and they require a room made especially for the device. In addition, the patient has to spend at least forty-five minutes inside the tube while the computer constructs images. It can be very uncomfortable for patients. I went inside an MRI tube one time just to try it, and it was miserable. The tube is almost right against your body. It can be very uncomfortable to sit in the tube for forty-five to sixty minutes. Also, some implanted electronic devices such as cardiac pacemakers and spinal cord stimulators are not MRI compatible.

There are now two types of MRIs. Due to the fact that the MRI is a closed imaging system and that it requires a long period of time, the open MRI was invented in the 2000s. The open MRI does not use a tube; instead; there is a big device that comes up against the body, and it is less irritating in terms of claustrophobia.

However, there is a significant problem with the open MRI: the quality of the image drops significantly in comparison to a closed MRI. A lot of the time, my patients request an open MRI because they have claustrophobia. I tell them that if they want me to assess their back condition in the best way, they need to find a way to tolerate the closed MRI so that I can get a clear image. If the patient moves inside the tube, the image becomes quite distorted, and all you end up with is a fuzzy picture, which is horrible and useless.

Sometimes I get referrals from chiropractors or physicians who automatically order an open MRI due to the fact that the patient requests it or because they do not want to bother the patient. When this occurs, sometimes I have to call them and request a closed MRI, especially when I am suspicious about some other pathology that I am having a difficult time viewing on the open MRI. Therefore, I urge the reader that, until the technology improves dramatically, it would be much more useful to get a closed MRI than an open MRI if you can tolerate it. It is not simply a matter of inconvenience but a matter of getting a full medical evaluation.

The next issue about MRIs is radiological reports. Once the image is complete, a radiologist reads the MRI and prepares a report. When patients see me, they have already read this report, and they have many questions regarding it. This creates a problem for me, because now I have to reassure the patients about something they have read in the MRI report that may not be important.

As a surgeon, I do not entirely rely on official radiological reports. I actually care little about radiological reports for two main reasons. Not to sound boastful, but I believe I do a better job than radiologists. Sometimes I get raised eyebrows when I make that statement. However, I have to say that all I do throughout the day, for every patient I see, is look at MRIs of the neck and the lower back. That is the bulk of what I do all day. A radiologist has to read many different images for many different conditions.

The second reason is that how a radiologist reads and interprets the image is very different from my read or a surgeon's interpretation. The radiologist is sitting in a room and going over image after image, for patient after patient, without any knowledge of what has happened to the person and what their complaint is. My normal practice is that, as I am talking to the patient and getting their history, I am reviewing the MRI. After that is done, I examine the patient. Following that, I review the MRI with the patient and go over all the findings to help them understand what is going on with them. After all, the most important factor in a first consultation is to make sure the patient understands what their situation is, and nothing is better than reviewing the actual MRI with the patient so they can understand and see the problem.

Sometimes I tell my patients that they need to bring their spouse at some point so they too can see the MRI and understand what the problem is with their family member. I believe it is very important for a spouse to understand and be involved in the process. When a person has a back condition, they are not sick or suffering from a medical condition in a way. The pain is very difficult to quantify or detect except in the person who is suffering from it. If back pain or neck pain turns into a chronic condition, this can put significant pressure on a relationship and can very easily affect a marriage. That is the reason I encourage my patients to bring their spouses to visits so that they can also understand what is going on. They do not have to come to every visit, but one visit to go over the MRI and see the problem is all I ask. Some people don't understand that even if you can smile or play golf, it does not mean that you don't have chronic pain.

As I said, a radiologist sits in some room and reviews the MRIs. They try to take note of what they think is unusual. However, as a surgeon, I am most interested in one aspect: what is causing my patient's pain and how it affects their quality of life. Patients come to me because they are suffering from a certain type of pain (back pain, neck pain, arm pain, or leg pain). After getting their history and performing a physical examination, I focus on a certain area that I believe is the culprit. I then come up with the appropriate treatment for that difficulty.

Sometimes the radiology report is challenging. I have to mention this because it is a big problem. There are two types of radiological reports. When a radiologist sees a disc herniation, they can use a measuring method to describe the problem. For example, they can say it is a 2 mm herniation at the level of L4-5 toward the right side, or about a 6 mm herniation at the level of L5-S1 in the midline. This is to give the surgeon the best idea of where and to what extent the problem is present based on careful measurement of the MRI. I really like this type of report because of its precision.

However, some radiologists use explanatory words to describe the problem. They use such words as "mild," "minimal," "moderate," and "severe." One of the issues with spine surgery is that in my world, looks do not matter. All day, I see patients that have very large problems and severe findings on an MRI. But these patients do well with some therapy, and their pain goes away, or their complaints are not very severe. On the other hand, I see patients that might have a 2–3 mm disc herniation, but they have severe symptoms to the point that they cannot even sit or stand for more than ten minutes. When a radiologist notes that an MRI shows "minimal herniation" or "moderate displacement" and somebody else reads the report, we might get the impression that the problem is not very big and the patient should not be suffering from a significant amount of pain. This creates a very significant problem in the way medicine is being practiced in the United States.

I try to do whatever I can to get a patient better without surgery. However, if all the treatments fail and the only option left is surgical intervention, the decision to proceed with the surgery is absolutely the patient's decision. They know how much pain they are in, and this is the life and the back that they have to live with. I have absolutely nothing to do with the decision of whether to proceed with surgery. My job is to listen to the patient and advise them on how I can help them or not, and to explain the surgical options, potential risks, and alternatives. I have many patients who are in severe pain, and they feel desperate and would like to proceed with surgery.

Here's the other problem. When a radiologist uses the words "mild displacement" or "minimal disc herniation" and I request surgery from an insurance company, the patient can be denied. This is a very unfortunate situation, because now the patient is suffering, and there is an appropriate medical treatment available to them, but they cannot get that simply because of a word the radiologist has chosen to describe the problem. This situation is frustrating for most surgeons, and there is nothing we can do about that. I really wish that the American Board of Radiology would instruct their radiologists to use measurement as interpretation in terms of millimeters as opposed to inappropriate or wrong descriptive words such as "minimal" or "moderate" when evaluating MRI images. If a radiologist calls it a 2 mm or 3 mm herniation, I know exactly what they are talking about. However, if the radiologist calls it "mild," that's hugely subjective. I have no idea what "mild" means to that person reading the MRI. Their definition of "mild" and my definition of "mild" may be completely different.

It is extremely important for the surgeon to review the actual films with the patient in detail. As a matter of fact, we have a big sign by our reception desk stating that every patient must bring their MRI with them. The presence of the actual MRI images is the most important aspect of the first visit with a patient. I tell my patients that the reason they are in my office is for me to examine them and go over the MRI with them so that they can better understand their condition as well as what could happen in their future. Overall, about 95 percent of the information I need to treat a patient comes from the medical history, clinical findings, and the MRI. The rest comes from X-rays and the CT scan. Imaging or electrophysiological studies can provide supportive or complementary information.

Disc Disease

Writing this book has brought up very interesting points for me and put a few things into perspective. The first commercially available MRI was in 1979. Therefore, the actual science of MRI is about as old as the movie *Saturday Night Fever*. When the young John Travolta was dancing around on the disco floor, this is about the time spine surgery was becoming a field. That does not leave us much time for developing our understanding of the spine. However, within this short time, we have made great advances.

The first condition I would like to discuss is damage to the intervertebral disc. As I mentioned earlier, the intervertebral disc is the cartilage between two vertebrae. The entire spine has an alternating structure of bone and intervertebral disc cartilage. The disc is composed of two sections: the mushy gelatinous center called *nucleus pulposus* and the very tough annular ring called the *annulus fibrosis*. This disc has two functions: stability, which means keeping the two bones together, and promoting motion. The disc achieves these goals through the spiral and interwoven collagen fibers in the annulus fibrosis. However, when the force that gets transmitted through this disc exceeds its threshold, the disc can get injured.

Before we go any further, the common name for this condition is *degenerative disc disease.* However, I truly believe this is a very old name that needs to be changed. It was first used when we had nothing but X-rays for evaluation of the spine. We called deterioration of the inter-vertebral discs "degenerative disc disease" without really knowing what was happening to the disc. Now that we have MRIs, we can actually eval-uate patients in a much earlier stage of disease, and we understand that these discs have sustained an injury. Therefore, it is more correctly called *damaged disc disease.*

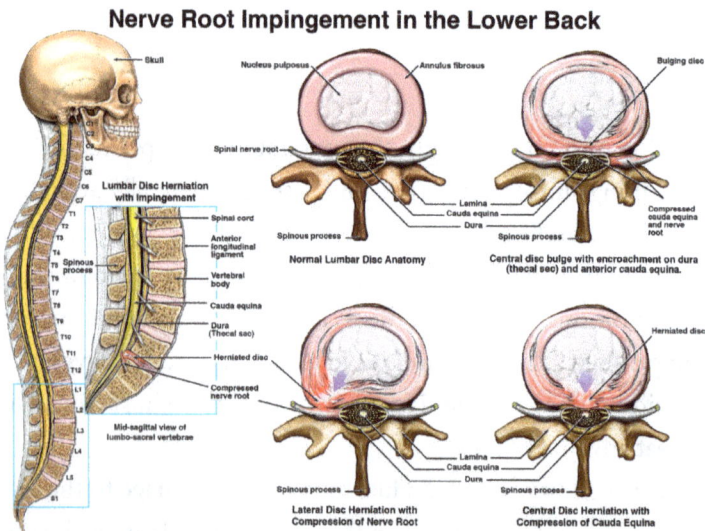

Figure 6: Nerve Root Impingement in the Lower Back

One of the most difficult problems when evaluating patients is that every person has a disc that is very special to that person in terms of its strength. Of course, different discs along the spine are exposed to dif-ferent levels of stress and forces. When a disc is injured, there can be spillage of the gelatinous core outside the boundary of the disc. This is called *disc herniation*. When the disc herniation is in the front or the side, it does not cause a significant problem. However, when the herniation is through the back, where the nerves are present, it can cause a significant problem.

The amount of slippage and the amount of material that spills out depends on the size of the tear. If the tear is very large, a large amount of the material can spill very quickly. However, if the tear is small, the spillage of gelatinous material can occur over months or even years. One of the most important things spine surgeons learn is that looks do not matter. That means that very bad-looking disc damage with a significant herniation can have low symptoms, or disc damage that is very minimally seen on an MRI can cause severe pain and discomfort.

As shown below in Figures 7 and 8, sometimes pain is manifest before an issue shows up on an MRI. In one case I worked on, a thirty-one-year-old patient was electrocuted, then fell ten feet to the ground. He injured his neck and lower back. He rated his neck pain at a seven on a one-to-ten scale, and his lower back pain at a nine. MRIs of his neck showed an obvious disc herniation at C5-6, but the lumbar spine MRI was negative for any problem, as shown in Figure 7. I recognized an abnormality at the L5-S1 disc, but I agreed with the radiologist that the finding was minimal. After an extensive workup, the patient decided to proceed with surgery. I told him that I could fix his neck because I was confident with the source of pain being C5-6, but I could not help him with his lower back pain because I was not confident where his pain was coming from. After a disc replacement in his cervical spine, his neck pain went away, but he continued to have lower back pain for another two years.

In Figure 8, an MRI taken two years later, it is now possible to clearly see a damaged disc at the L5-S1 level. This is a good example of a patient who had sustained an injury to his lower back and was in severe pain, yet the initial MRI did not show any damage.

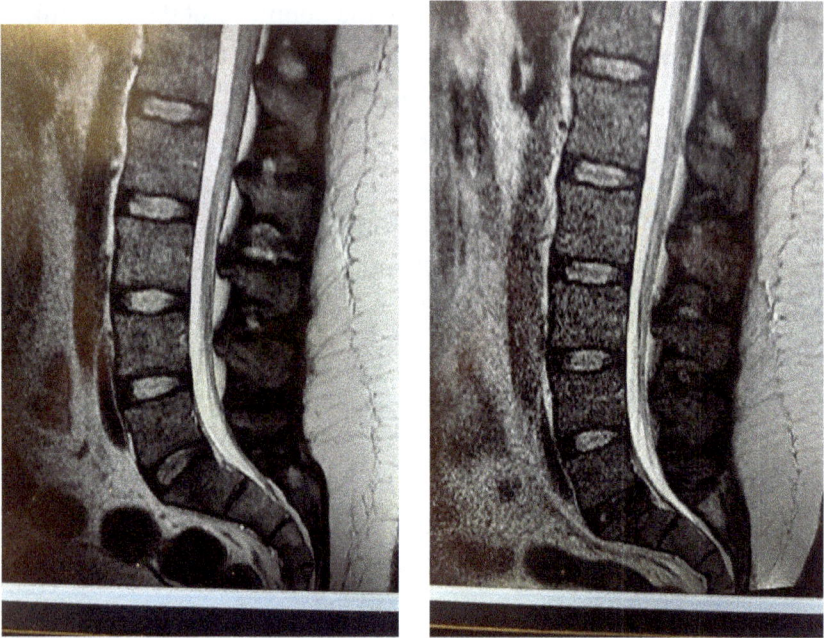

Figure 7 (left): A Thirty-One-Year-Old Man Complained about Back Pain for Two Years. Initial MRI Was Negative. Figure 8 (right): Subsequent MRI Two Years Later Showed Damage at Lower Disc.

In 2014, I had a forty-eight-year-old female patient who had been suffering from severe neck pain, headaches, and left arm pain for about three years. She stated that she had been able to tolerate the pain for the first couple of years. But, in the year prior to seeing me, the pain had become unbearable and had begun affecting every aspect of her life. She had tried multiple sessions of physical therapy, as well as two epidural injections, as well as radiofrequency ablation, to no avail. She even had Botox injections. She was sitting in my office crying.

There was clearly a problem with her, but her MRI report was negative, at least according to the radiologist. I remember that the radiologist had looked at every disc and stated they were all within normal limits. In their impression of the report, the radiologist read it as being a normal cervical spine. As a spine surgeon, I could see an abnormality and bulge at the level of C5-6. The patient's symptoms were also consistent with a damaged disc at the level of C5-6. However, the abnormality was not remarkable. In a way, I was not upset at the radiologist and understood his evaluation. Sometimes a spine surgeon has the upper hand in reading the MRI, as they get to talk to the patient and perform an examination.

I followed this patient for about six months and sent her to obtain another series of epidural and Botox injections. I also sent her to see a neurologist in my building. The Botox injections helped but not significantly. At her fifth visit, she was in tears again and said she did not want to continue living like this. We continued all the possible treatments, including narcotics, muscle relaxants, and nerve stabilizers. She tried a nerve stimulator known as a TENS unit and everything we could think of. I eventually told her that I had tried everything and there was nothing that could be done for her. This caused significant grief. I also advised her that I would refer her to a pain specialist, and I encouraged her to get a second opinion.

Practicing in a small town, just like everything else in life, has its positives and negatives. The positive is that you get to know everyone and can make a good reputation in town very quickly. The negative is that you can quickly get a poor reputation if you do not do a good job. In addition, there is a very good chance your patient is related to somebody on staff, another patient, or possibly a neighbor. That makes it difficult to turn somebody away. But I had run out of tests to order for this patient and had run out of treatments to offer her. I truly did not have anything else.

Unfortunately, because of her negative MRI report, no other surgeons were even willing to see her, so she came back to see me again. This time she said I was her last and only hope. She felt I knew what was wrong with her and what could be done for her, and she was right. I knew it was the C5-6 disc that was bothering her. The solution for this was an anterior cervical discectomy and fusion. I was very honest with her that the condition was not very obvious on the MRI. I would be a hero if surgery made her better, but I would be in trouble if she was not better with surgery. In fact, I told her that if it failed, I could be reported to the American Board of Orthopaedic Surgery and could possibly be accused of committing malpractice as well as unethical practices. She told me she would sign any paper stating it was her decision and that I had warned her against the surgery, to get the responsibility off me so she could have the surgery. I explained to the patient that I could understand her thinking, but she might not remember this conversation if something went wrong. After a very lengthy conversation, I agreed to proceed with the surgery.

Fortunately, there is a very good ending to this story. I performed a one-level anterior cervical discectomy and fusion, and all her pain resolved. (See Figure 9 below.) She was very thankful, and she told me that I changed her life.

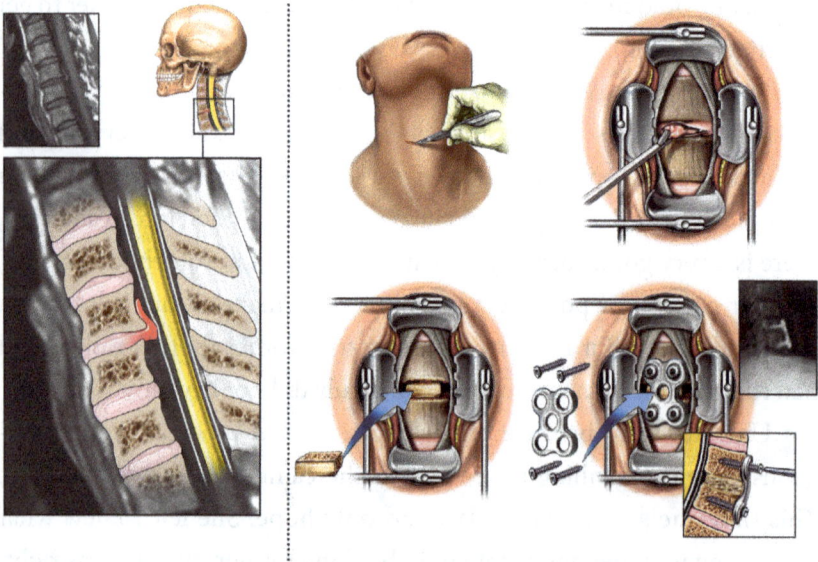

Figure 9: Cervical Disc Herniation with Surgical
Discectomy and Fusion Surgery

Overall, in my practice, I have operated on six patients that had a negative MRI report. The goal of these two stories is to show that what appears on the MRI has nothing to do with the amount of pain a patient is suffering from. We truly do not understand the pain pathways, but we know pain has to do with inflammation. At this point, there is no method to see where the inflammation is present or to detect where the pain molecules are present. There is research being done to find a marker in blood that indicates if a patient has pain. Truthfully, I am baffled by this. We as surgeons don't need blood tests; we need imaging studies. We should stop trying to figure out if a patient is being truthful and start believing our patients. If we don't believe our patients, we certainly cannot treat them.

My treatment of a very healthy fifty-one-year-old nurse is another good case in point. While trying to help a patient, the nurse fell down, causing him severe lower back and right leg pain. I followed his case for about a year and a half and was involved from the beginning of his care. I sent him for epidural steroid injections, facet blocks, radiofrequency ablation, etc. He stated that his pain was so severe that he could not work anymore. He was working modified duty as a nurse in a supervisor position. However, even that position was becoming difficult. I found it very admirable that he was working through this pain. However, he broke down in front of me and started crying. He stated that he could not live with the pain anymore. He had tried everything and had lost the weight I advised him to lose, but he was still in miserable pain. He followed all my recommendations. At that point, the phone calls started coming in. His primary care physician and his chiropractor started calling me and sending me e-mails. They, too, were very upset with my patient's symptoms. They had already done all that they could and were looking to me for the next step.

I had a video meeting with his primary care physician to go over the MRI. I explained that it looked very benign and that I could not identify where his pain was coming from. I explained that as a last resort, we could do a procedure called *discography*. Discography is a test to detect where the pain is coming from and can be done for the cervical spine and the lumbar spine. During the procedure, the patient is completely awake. We cannot give them pain medicine because we want to know where the pain is coming from, so stopping the pain would defeat the whole purpose of the exercise. Under X-ray, long needles are inserted into the discs. Once the position of the needles is confirmed using anterior, posterior, and lateral X-rays, we inject a combination of saline and radiopaque solution into the disc.

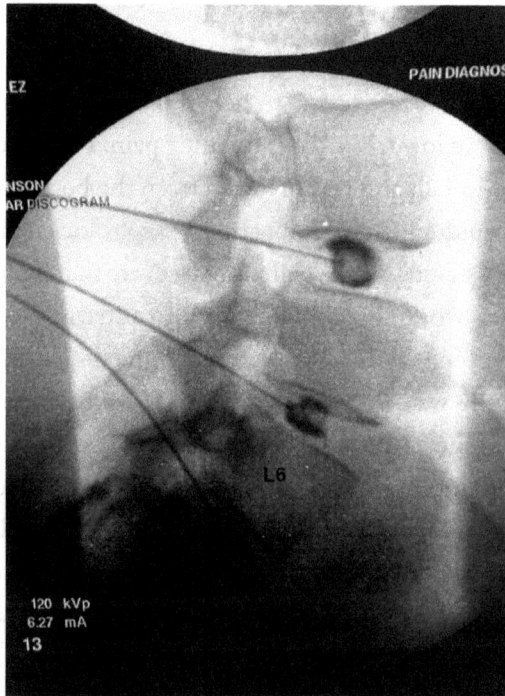

Figure 10: Discography Example

The goal is to pressurize and stimulate the disc to see if we can identify the disc that is causing the problem. The patient is covered with a cloth, and they do not know which disc is being injected. If we inject a good disc and see the distribution of dye is good and the patient has no symptoms, then that disc is not the source of the pain. However, if we inject a disc and they have pain, we ask them if this is the pain they came to see me for. If they answer yes, then we have a positive finding. It would also confirm the test if the distribution of dye shows damage to the disc and a tear in the annulus.

I offered my nurse-patient this test, and he accepted without hesitation. I advised him that the test would likely be painful, and he did not care. He said if there was a procedure to find out the cause of his pain, he would do it tomorrow. I sent him for the discography.

Unfortunately, the results were confusing. First, the needle could not be threaded to the L5-S1 disc. The L4-5 disc was found to be a source of pain, and I was assured that the disc at the level of L4-5 was the pain generator by the doctor who did the test. However, for some reason, I was not convinced.

Each description of pain location, radiation of pain, or the behavior of pain is a clue for me. Due to the fact that I do not have a physician assistant in my practice and my patients see me personally each time they come to my office, I have compiled a significant amount of data over the years in terms of the behavior of each condition. Somehow, this time my intuition was not in tune with the L4-5 disc being the problem.

The phone calls started coming again from the chiropractor and the primary care physician asking, "Now what?" After the discography, I had to tell the patient that I could not do surgery, as I really did not think I could help him. He began crying and stated he would try anything if there were hope that he could be fixed. I told him that I had already tried everything and still could not pinpoint the source of his pain to fix it. I told him as a last resort, I would repeat the discography with somebody I trust who is extremely good at these. The patient agreed. That indicated how much pain he was suffering from, as he did not argue about undergoing a second discography; it is a very painful procedure. I had not believed he would go for that, but he was eager. I sent him to my trusted doctor.

This time, the results were positive at the level of L5-S1. All along, I had suspected that it was the L5-S1 disc causing the patient's pain. He did experience pain at that level, but the dye distribution was actually in the pattern of a normal disc.

Now I had a patient crying in my office who had already seen me at least ten times, as well as a chiropractor and primary care physician who kept calling me. I also had an inconclusive discography and another discography that showed that the disc at L5-S1 was causing pain but that the injury could not be confirmed. In addition, the MRI did not show anything. I explained to him that I did not want to perform surgery because I was unable to determine where the pain was coming from with high confidence. He was distraught and asked if there was anything else that could be done. I told him that, unfortunately, he would have to live like this. He told me he could not live like this, and this could not be his life. I considered sending him to a psychiatrist to receive medicine for depression. He had accepted my treatment plan to this point, but he asked how an antidepressant medicine could possibly take away his pain. Truthfully, I did not have an answer for him.

I told him that I was certain it was the L5-S1 disc causing his low back pain. However, the evidence was not strong. To proceed with surgery, a greater level of confidence is necessary, which was not present in his case. He stated that even if there was only a 10 percent chance of getting better, he wanted to take the chance. I told him my job is not to deny him treatment that could potentially help him. I had the same kind of conversation with him that I had with the patient in my previous example: I told the nurse the surgery could put my entire practice in danger. If this case was put before an orthopedic board, it would fail me on the spot because it is a bad treatment plan for a spine surgeon. I would fail another surgeon if he went forward with a surgery like this. I had an extensive conversation with his primary care physician and his chiropractor, and they understood the predicament I was in.

Long story short, I could not live with myself knowing that I could help him and did not. Therefore, I proceeded with a one-level anterior and posterior L5-S1 fusion. It was a big surgery. I went through the abdomen, sweeping the abdominal contents to the side, removing the disc, replacing it with a prosthesis, going through the back, and fusing from the back.

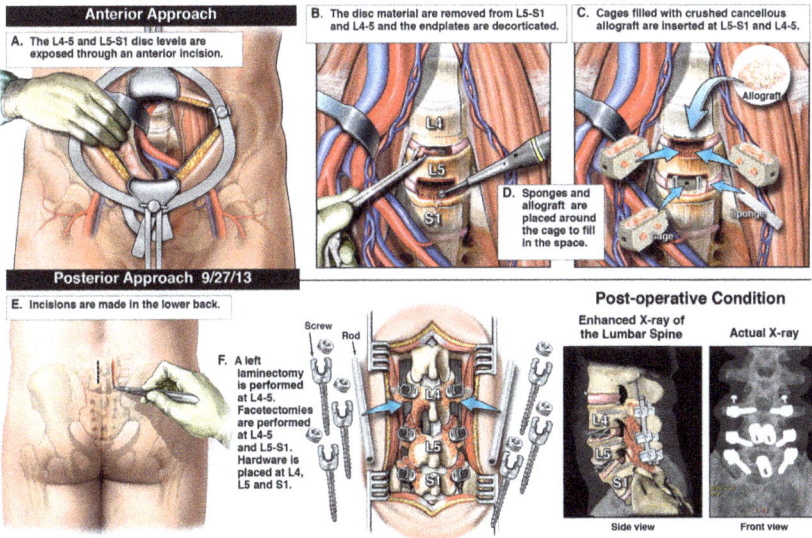

Figure 11: L4-5 and L5-S1 Lumbar Spine Anterior and Posterior Surgeries

I will never forget the smile on his face in the recovery room after surgery. As soon as I walked in and saw his face, I knew he was going to be fine and that we did the right surgery. This was a truly triumphant moment for me.

However, this does not mean that any patient suffering from back pain with a negative MRI should run to the closest spine surgeon and demand surgical intervention. With these two cases, I had a good idea where the pain was coming from in spite of the imaging studies. There is a huge difference between these scenarios. I do not want to give the impression that people who suffer from back pain with a negative MRI study should demand surgery. On the other hand, I truly believe there are a lot of patients who are suffering from severe pain and do have a problem. Unfortunately for some of them, the MRI does not pick it up or does not show that it is bad enough for the surgeon to risk a potentially inappropriate surgery.

This is not a situation I like to face in my practice. With each of the patients who had minimal findings that I have performed surgery for, I have lost a significant amount of sleep and have developed a stomach ulcer. These two cases are the exception, not the rule. These are just the patients that I knew I could help, even though their imaging studies were not very obvious. I have had many patients that I have told I cannot perform surgery, and that was it.

My patients always ask me what they can do to get better if they have pain due to a damaged disc. They have been told that they need to do certain exercises or follow a certain diet. The obvious things include weight control, changing bad habits, and having a healthy diet, but not much else can really be done. We do not understand why the majority of people with an injury get better with some therapy, while a small percentage do not get better and end up needing surgery. Some people respond to steroid injections, whereas other people do not at all. Some people with a bad-looking disc herniation might have minimal pain, while other people with minimal MRI findings might have severe pain.

One thing is for sure. Lifting is the activity that is going to damage discs or aggravate existing conditions. The force of lifting an object goes right through the injured disc. Here's why: The spine supports the upper trunk and whatever you're lifting. These discs are between the bones, so when weight is lifted, the force travels right through the disc.

I sometimes get into arguments with therapists about this topic. Their advice is to strengthen the core muscles. I totally agree with the idea that strengthening the core muscles is very important for balance and the well-being of the spine. However, muscles do not support weight. Even if the muscles supporting the spine are very strong, once you lift weight, it goes entirely through the disc. Therefore, strengthening the paraspinal muscles is not a green light to lift heavy weights. I advise my patients to avoid lifting heavy weight. Of course, the amount of weight can differ for different conditions and different individuals. In addition, there could be a delay between the activity of lifting and the resurgence of pain. You can be pain-free for two to three days after lifting a couch , then cough or sneeze and end up with severe pain lasting a week or two. I see a lot of patients that say they were not doing anything at all and just woke up with the pain. I tell them that if they go back two to three days, they would probably find an activity that started the cascade of inflammation that resulted in their pain.

The technique of lifting is very important as well. If you bend forward and lift an object with your back, you are more prone to injury than if you squat down, keep your back straight, and use your legs to lift the weight.

More About Facet Joints

Facet joints are not very well understood in the world of spine surgery. As I discussed in Chapter One, "Anatomy of the Spine," each vertebra has two processes that extend up and connect with the two processes that extend downward. These processes, from the vertebrae above and below, form a facet joint.

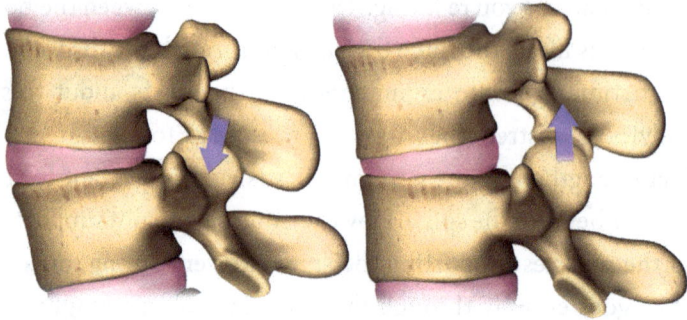

Figure 12: Facet Joints in Motion

These are gliding surfaces that are covered by hyaline cartilage. This is the same cartilage that we have in other joints in our body, such as the knee, shoulder, and knuckles. This joint has a capsule with fluid for lubrication inside, just like any other joint.

We know that facet joints have a very important function. The most efficient way of creating stability in a three-dimensional manner is to have at least three points of contact. This happens in the spine. One point of contact is the intervertebral disc, and the other two points of contact are facet joints, one on each side when you look from the back. Studies done in the early 1970s showed that loss of these facet joints causes significant instability in that segment of the spine. We know that their function is very important and, as surgeons, we do whatever we can to preserve the facet joints.

It is very difficult to determine what percentage of facet pain contributes to overall neck or back pain. Anything that moves in the body and has a significant innervation (which facet joints do) can break down and can cause pain. This condition is called *facet syndrome*. Because the disc and the two facet joints move together and form one unit, when one goes bad, then chances are the others go bad as well. Therefore, it is extremely difficult to differentiate how much pain is coming from which part. No one is actively working to answer that question because the treatment for a damaged disc and the treatment for a painful facet joint are often the same: fuse the two bones and eliminate the motion in that area.

As I said, the facet joints contribute significantly to the stability of the motion segment. The other very important factor is that the facet joint orientation can tell us quite a bit about what type of motion that segment goes through. For example, in the cervical spine, facet joints are more horizontal than in the rest of the spine. This tells you that the segments in the cervical spine have a much better range of motion, which is obvious because the head has to move around quite a bit. We know the range of motion of the neck is higher than that of the lower back. In the lower back, facet joints are more vertical, which adds significantly to translational stability. A vertically oriented facet joint does not allow one vertebra to slip over the other vertebra. This orientation adds more stability in terms of moving back and forth, which is extremely important in the lumbar spine. Motion of a vertebra in the lumbar spine over the vertebra below is a rotational motion. Facet joints only allow a rotational motion of one vertebra over the other in the lumbar spine. I will allude to this very important point in Chapters Five, Six, and Seven.

Due to the fact that the facet joints in the cervical spine are more horizontal, it only makes sense that they contribute more in terms of carrying weight than other parts of the spine. That means the discs in the lumbar spine get the brunt of the stress and weight that is being carried through that segment. This leads me to believe that facet syndrome should be more prevalent in the cervical spine as opposed to the lumbar spine. However, this is a topic I have not yet studied in detail.

Facet syndrome is a painful facet, and we believe it is caused by an inflammatory process and is connected to disc incompetence. Once the disc gets injured, it cannot hold weight or function very well. Therefore, some of that stress gets transferred to the facet joints, and they start wearing down. At what point the facet becomes painful is very difficult to determine. However, an acute event such as trauma or a car accident can contribute and cause facet joints to become painful.

The treatment for facet syndrome is often facet joint injection. This procedure is done either under fluoroscopy, which uses X-rays, or ultrasound imaging to pass a needle down to the facet joint and inject it with numbing medication and anti-inflammatory cortisone. This is done on both sides due to the fact that if one facet has been injured, the chances are that the other facet has been injured as well.

It is very difficult to determine if the patient's pain is coming from the facets or the disc at one motion segment. However, one test that can theoretically give us some sort of an idea is what we call an extension test. I ask the patient to stand up, and I place one hand on their chest and the other on their back. I gently push on their chest to bend them backward. This jams the facet joints by hyperextending them. If this maneuver causes the back pain to reoccur, then it could be facet-generated pain. However, this test is not accurate and only gives us an idea of what may be going on. It is important to keep in mind tha,t at this time, we have absolutely no way of knowing how much facet joint pain is contributing to the overall back or neck pain.

Spinal Stenosis

Spinal stenosis means tightness of the central canal. It can present as back pain or leg pain, either bilateral or unilateral. A typical complaint of spinal stenosis is pain with ambulation. When the patient walks a distance, the pain comes on in their back and radiates into their bilateral buttocks and down their legs. However, when the patient rests, the pain gets a lot better. This happens because the nerves that are traversing the central canal get pinched.

Spinal stenosis is mostly caused by disc deterioration over time and comes on mostly with age. Once a disc deteriorates at a level, it starts settling. As it settles, the facet joints get overworked, and they start becoming arthritic and bigger. The ligaments in the back of the spine that are nice and tight initially will loosen like a curtain coming down.

The combination of a settled disc, hypertrophied facet joints, and ligaments intruding into the canal causes tightness of the central canal and impingement of the nerves that are passing through the canal. This mostly happens in the lower lumbar region, commonly at the level of L4-5. However, it can happen at multiple levels.

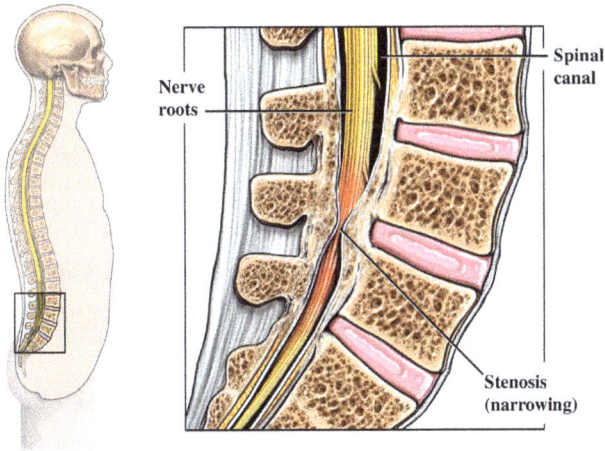

Figure 13: Spinal Stenosis

A patient can go on with this problem for many years when the condition is stable, but the problem can deteriorate quickly. The first step is physical therapy and chiropractic care. The next step is steroid injections. The last step is surgery. In the initial phase of this condition, physical therapy and chiropractic care are usually very successful in treating the symptoms. As the condition progresses, epidural injections become very successful in controlling the pain. However, for some people, steroid injections are not successful, and we have to intervene surgically.

The condition is easy to diagnose because you can see a pinched nerve on the MRI, but surgical treatment is very difficult. The surgery for this condition involves unroofing the canal and decompressing the nerves. In addition to decompression of the central canal, sometimes we have to fuse that level to stabilize the spine. The decision to fuse or not to fuse is a much-debated topic in the world of spine surgery, and I will not get into that here because it is too technical. I will say that due to the fact that you have to remove a significant amount of bone to decompress the nerves in advanced cases, you are committed to fusing and stabilizing that area.

Sacroiliac Joint Pain

Sacroiliac joint pain is one of the most mysterious conditions in the spine. It is a condition that originates from the sacroiliac joint, between the sacrum and iliac bones on each side. This joint is part of the pelvis, but it has been treated by spine surgeons because it is part of the complex of lower back pain.

We do not understand to what extent sacroiliac joint pain contributes to the overall number of lower back pain conditions. Surgeons are sharply divided in terms of determining its contribution to lower back pain syndrome. Some surgeons believe there are a very small number of people who suffer from this pain. Another group of surgeons believes there is a significant contribution from the sacroiliac joint to overall lower back pain syndrome.

The sacroiliac joint is a very stable joint. It is not like other joints that move freely, are covered with hyaline cartilage, and have a capsule. The sacroiliac joint does have an area of cartilage; however, the majority of it is composed of thick fibrous structures that hold the sacrum and ilium tightly together. This is mostly a nonfunctioning joint. In anatomy labs, when we examine the sacroiliac joints, we quickly realize it takes a significant amount of force to get the joints to move. I believe its function is to dissipate the forces in the pelvis and make the pelvis more resilient against fractures by allowing micromotion between the bones. In addition, in females, there has to be a mechanism allowing the pelvis to open

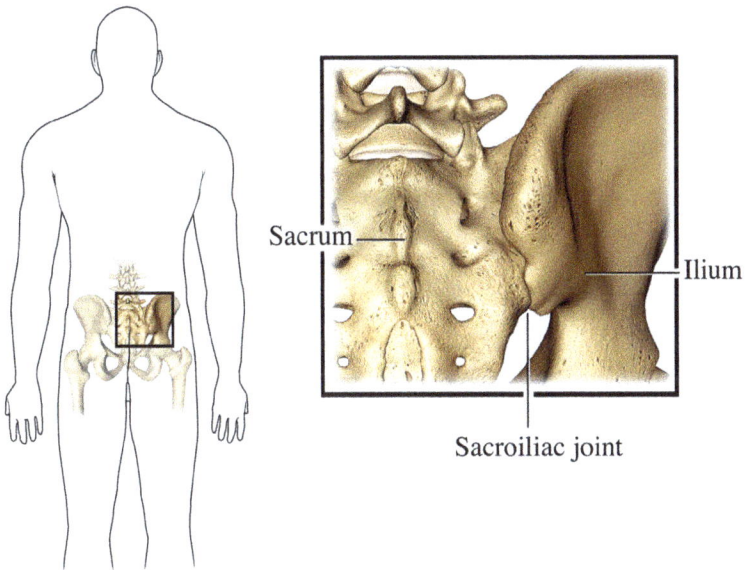

Sacrum

Ilium

Sacroiliac joint

Figure 14: Sacroiliac Joint

up to allow for childbirth. Under the effect of certain hormones excreted during childbirth, the anterior symphysis pubis and sacroiliac ligaments loosen and allow for the pelvic bone to stretch open.

It is very difficult to describe the symptoms of sacroiliac joint pain. In my practice, I am always alert for pain that is over the sacroiliac joint in the right or left buttock area. This is mostly a dull, achy pain rather than a sharp, stabbing pain. The treatment for this condition is physical therapy, stretching exercises, and steroid injections in the sacroiliac joint. The very last option is the fusion of the joint.

There are other conditions of the spine that can cause pain, including tumors, infections, metabolic bone disease, and others. While I deal with such issues in my medical practice, they are relatively rare compared to herniated discs and spinal stenosis and are therefore beyond the scope of this book.

CHAPTER THREE

Nonoperative Treatments for Neck and Back Pain

PART I: MANIPULATIVE TREATMENTS

In general, I divide the treatment of neck and lower back pain into three stages. The first stage is called *manipulative treatments*. In this stage, the idea is to manipulate the body externally and try to eliminate the neck and back pain. This category, a world in itself, includes physical therapy, chiropractic care, acupuncture, massage therapy, yoga, etc. The second stage is what I call *therapeutic pain procedures*, which include injections. Both of those stages are the main topics of this chapter. The third stage is a surgical intervention to which I devote all of Chapter Four.

Even though I make my living as a spine surgeon, my actual job is to avoid surgical intervention. However, if nonoperative care fails to control a patient's pain to a tolerable degree, surgical intervention is indicated.

I have a unique practice. Most spine surgeons in private practice only do surgery. Very early in my practice, I realized that was not going to satisfy my appetite for progress. I did not want to be a technician only; I wanted to contribute to my field. I could not have done that in an academic setting. It's hard to explain, but I am a free thinker and could not conform to a mold. I had to find a way to contribute on my terms and at my own pace. As mentioned, I am heavily involved with research and development, and very involved with nonoperative care. I am very familiar with pain procedures and perform some of them myself. Therefore, I have extensive experience with early stages of spine conditions as opposed to being the last guy who sees the patient.

The decision of whether to do surgery is the patient's. In my practice, I recommend surgery in the case of a herniated disc that is causing spinal cord impingement. Unfortunately, the spinal cord is not a structure that can recover from compression easily. Most of the time, the injury that the spinal cord sustains due to external pressure is irreversible. That is why, in the world of spine surgery, we tend to intervene surgically when we see spinal cord symptoms. The whole idea is to decompress the spinal cord so we can preserve its function. Occasionally, I see a patient who is not really suffering from neck pain; however, they have dysfunction of their spinal cord because of a large disc. I must explain to these patients that with a fairly large-sized surgery to decompress the spinal cord, it may be hard to see the true benefit of the surgery. The "benefit" is that it will stop their spinal cord from deteriorating and getting worse.

The bad news is that neck and back pain is extremely common. The exact incidence of neck and back pain is debatable, and there are lots of different estimates, but it is very common. The good news is that most people who suffer from neck or back pain get better with proper, appropriately timed, nonoperative care. I tell my patients that I only end up doing surgery on a minimal number of patients that come to see me. Between 90 to 95 percent of the time, I can help patients control pain with appropriate nonoperative care.

I know that the idea of surgery can be highly seductive. A patient can imagine being wheeled into the operating room and being rid of their intractable pain a few hours later. Unlike physical therapy, yoga, or other exercise routines, which all require some serious effort—sometimes quite strenuous—and discipline, surgery sounds like a great passive option. Let me disabuse you of that notion. It is a team effort to have a successful surgical outcome. I always tell my patients that when I plan to operate, we are in it together.

There is nothing worse in my world than a patient who does not get better with surgery. When a patient does not improve after an operation, we do not just walk away and completely forget about their situation. I do not discharge a patient from my practice until I know I have done everything I can. If the patient does not improve, I have to start from zero with a complete reevaluation. The biggest reason for that is because there are plenty of times a patient might have a simple problem after surgery that can easily be corrected. However, when a patient is discharged from a surgeon's practice, the next doctor might never address those issues.

One of the most common reasons for a patient's pain not going away after surgery is painful hardware. The screws I place inside a patient's body are huge, and sometimes the sheer size of the screws causes significant pain. Postoperative pain due to hardware is widespread. In this case, the treatment is straightforward. We can remove the hardware, and that can reduce the postoperative pain significantly.

A difficult problem after surgery is to determine if the fusion is solid or not. I have many patients who come to see me as a second opinion, and I determine that they have an unfused or unhealed surgery. Unfortunately, in these situations, I have to repeat the surgery and try to get them to heal. However, if the patient is discharged from a surgeon's practice and ends up in pain management, they might be suffering from back pain for the rest of their lives without anyone knowing the cause of it.

When I tell my patients that surgery is teamwork, I explain that I have to do my part and they have to do their part. That might be anything from weight loss to a healthy diet to routine exercise, and sometimes it means major changes in their life. Sometimes I must tell my patients that their job is too strenuous and that it is prudent for them to change their job. The goal of the surgery is not to give them a brand-new back, but to let them get a good night's sleep or take just one-third of the medicine that they normally require. Spine surgery is a field in which we keep the bar high, and our goal should be to eliminate the pain for our patients. However, at the same time, we need to make our patients understand that they should not have unrealistic expectations of recovery and results. Therefore, I would like to make an important point that surgery is not effortless on the patient's side at all. As a matter of fact, sometimes it means a lifelong commitment to protecting the surgery so that the results can last them a lifetime.

I had dinner with a friend who was a board-certified neurologist. Toward the end of the dinner at his home, he asked my opinion about his wife. She was suffering from lower back and left leg pain. She had tried physical therapy and two injections with no results. I spoke to his wife and looked at the MRI. She had a huge disc herniation at L4-5, completely pinching the L5 nerve root on the left side. I told my friend that she would benefit from surgery and that this is a very successful surgery.

He proceeded to say that there was no way he would allow that to happen. He said they had seen a spine surgeon in New York already who recommended surgery; however, he was not comfortable with his wife undergoing surgery. I asked him what his rationale was. He told me that he hears from radiologist colleagues who review X-rays, MRIs, and CT scans all day for patients who have had failed back surgery. That is when it hit me. I explained to my friend that most patients do get better with spine surgery, but he would not have heard about that aspect of spine surgery because those patients do not require additional MRIs or other imaging studies. We do imaging studies only for patients who are not doing well.

About two months later, his wife could not bear the pain anymore, and she underwent a one-level lumbar laminectomy and discectomy. I saw them six months later; his wife said that the surgery had changed her life and she was very happy.

That interaction taught me something: It is much better not to ask a specialist what they think of another specialty. If someone tries a treatment modality offered by a specialist and they get better, they will not seek other specialists. However, if they do not get better, they start seeking alternative treatments and other physicians. As a spine surgeon, I see patients all day who have had other treatments and did not get better. We all have a personal bias based on our limited experience.

Chiropractic Care

One of the physical rehab techniques that I really like is chiropractic care. In 2005, a patient named Daniel came to see me for consultation. Daniel was a seventy-eight-year-old gentleman who was suffering from significant lower back pain for about two years. When he saw me, he had already completed an entire course of physical therapy and had already tried steroid injections in the lower back. Despite these treatments, his pain remained very debilitating. Daniel told me that his life quality was poor, and he could not get a good night's sleep night after night.

After taking his history and performing a physical examination, I reviewed his MRI with him. All the discs in the lumbar spine were worn out. He had bone-on-bone contact in three discs in the lower back, and the other two discs were not that great either. That means there was no cushion left between the vertebrae. He was experiencing sharp, stabbing pain that turned into a burning sensation. This started in his lower back and radiated into his buttocks and down both legs.

This was a very difficult visit. As a spine surgeon, I am the last stop. When a patient comes to see me, they have completed what we call *nonoperative treatment*. They are expecting and, in most cases, hoping for some sort of surgical intervention. They must be in quite a bit of pain to come to a surgeon for a consultation.

Typically, I divide my patients into two categories: simple and complex. A simple case has one or two bad discs. A complex case has three or more discs that are injured. Another way of explaining it is to say that there are two types of patients. One type has a problem in a localized area, and the other type has a problem that has spread over a wide region. Patients who fall into the simple category with an injured disc in a specific area do very well with surgery. There is a very sharp boundary between where they have a problem and where their back is healthy. The success rate for these patients is very high and at almost 90 percent. These are the patients who make our job fun. They are happy and appreciative, and we feel good about ourselves as surgeons.

However, a patient in the complex category with three or more bad discs has a problem that is not limited to a specific area. Treatment is very challenging in these patients, and sometimes this can give an undeserved bad reputation to spine surgery. I explain to these patients that the most important aspect is information. The more informed the patient is, the better the outcome gets. These patients need to understand exactly what goes through the surgeon's mind and why he decided to perform a certain procedure. I review their MRIs with them at every single visit. These patients might require multiple surgeries throughout their lifetime.

In this group of patients, sometimes the surgery must be staged. In this case, the notion of multiple surgeries is not bad. I tell my patient that if I do one large surgery, and God forbid things do not go well and they continue to have significant symptoms, it is challenging to try to figure out what went wrong or what the problem is. However, suppose I break the large surgery up into two stages of surgery. In that case, I have a much better chance of discovering problems as I go along and therefore have an opportunity to solve them.

I had a very long discussion with Daniel. I explained in detail the surgery that he needed and went over the steps we had to take. He needed a five-level fusion with twelve screws and two rods—a massive and risky procedure. I told him that he should not have the surgery and that if he were my father, I would advise him not to go ahead. However, it was his decision, and I would not deny him surgery that could potentially help him. He looked dejected.

I explained to Daniel that the other goal of surgery with this magnitude of difficulty was to stabilize the pain, not necessarily eliminate the pain. Sometimes I tell patients that the notion of failed back surgery is not fair. Many times, surgery accomplishes an important milestone that the patient unfortunately cannot appreciate: a stabilization of the back so that the pain does not get worse. That is a very important topic that needs to be explained to a patient preoperatively. I spent some time with Daniel and talked about his activities and activity modification.

It is extremely difficult to tell a patient that there is nothing I can do for them and tell them that they are stuck with the pain for the rest of their life. In twenty years of practice, I have not found a good way to tell this to a patient without making them very upset. These situations take a toll on me as well. I feel inadequate, and I feel bad. When I started my practice, I was warned by my professors that I need to be careful with these complex situations. I wanted to be a healer and make a difference for patients who are desperate. In a good portion of the first part of my practice, I performed these complex surgeries, and I did get some good results. However, I learned very quickly and realized what my professors had been trying to tell me. Even worse than telling a patient that they will have to deal with their situation for the rest of their life is to have a patient who has not gotten better after you have operated on them. That situation is devastating to a surgeon, and that is what you learn in your practice as a spine surgeon. It takes decades to learn to approach these problems with extreme caution. When I tell a patient that there is nothing I can do for them in surgery, they just do not want to leave the office. They cannot understand in that thirty-minute visit that they are out of options.

During the first part of my career, I practiced in a small town in California called Yuba City, with a population of 45,000 people. It also covered a vast surrounding area, but the city itself was very small. That meant that if I went to a local store, there would be a very good chance that I would bump into a patient I had performed surgery on. In the case of Daniel, I was in the emergency room attending an emergency call two years later when I bumped into him. He recognized me, and I recognized him. I asked him how he was doing because I was very curious. He had a smile on his face. He told me that after I talked to him, he consulted with three other surgeons. He gave me the names of local surgeons in Sacramento who are very good, established surgeons. They had told him the same thing that I told him. Those surgeons agreed that he needed a five-level fusion, and they recommended against proceeding with surgery.

While going through these second opinions, Daniel stated that he spoke to a friend who recommended a chiropractor in town. The chiropractor had a traction decompressive machine. For this treatment, the patient lays on the table with one strap on the chest and one on the pelvis. The straps are connected to a pulley that applies traction using a computerized program. This device tries to stretch the lumbar or cervical spine. The idea is that the inflammation, which causes pain, creates scar formation. With scar formation, there is more inflammation and a very vicious cascade resulting in contractures, scars, and pain. The whole idea is to decompress the area, allow the site to calm down, and decrease the inflammation. Daniel informed me that he tried six to ten sessions of traction decompressive treatments of the lumbar spine, and his pain went away completely. He was very happy, and he was very happy with me for my honesty and the time I spent with him.

It is difficult to know how many Daniels are out there, but stories like Daniel's have made me very interested in chiropractic care. In spine surgery, I learn from everybody, including professors in major universities, my colleagues, my patients, and even from my mother. Daniel's story had the absolute best ending and taught me quite a bit. Just like any other nonoperative care, traction decompressive treatment has successes and failures. Over the following decade, I befriended chiropractors and learned quite a bit from them. This greatly helped me treat the patients in my practice.

When a patient initially experiences neck or back pain, they often go to different providers seeking help. Most people go to their primary care physician. That is because they think their condition can get better with a symptom-relieving medicine, though not necessarily narcotics. Unfortunately, there is no good medicine to treat neck or lower back pain. The way that health care is set up, you have to see your primary care physician first, and they provide referrals to the necessary providers. If a patient sees their primary care physician and does not improve with helpful medicine, they usually get referred to physical therapy.

Another group of people go to their local chiropractor to seek care, or it could be a combination of physical therapy and chiropractic care. The most common question I get asked is, between the two, which one is better? I like chiropractic care more for the spine; let me explain.

My residency and fellowship training taught me that chiropractic care and physical therapy are not very helpful. After I finished my fellowship, I was approached by a group of surgeons in Yuba City, forty-five minutes north of Sacramento, that was looking for an orthopedic spine surgeon to join their practice; I took the job. Coming from Boston and New York, I had difficulty adjusting to a small town. I saw the position as temporary and gave myself one or two years to relocate. I had never thought I would practice in a small town and saw myself in a major city near a major hospital.

I have been through a lot of adversity in my life. I have learned that sometimes when you are very upset about something and wish it never happened, it might turn out to be the best thing that ever happened to you. Such was the case with my decision to practice in a small town. In retrospect, moving to Yuba City was the best thing that could have happened to me in my career.

In a small town, there is only one of every store, including one Walmart, one Home Depot, etc. When patronizing these stores in town,

I often saw one of my patients or perhaps one of their family members or a referring physician. My patients were also very close friends with my staff, who lived in the same town. My staff also encountered patients or their relatives around town almost every day. There were good and bad aspects about this. The bad aspect was that any bad result would spread through town very quickly. I was the only orthopedic spine surgeon in town, and the other neurosurgeon in town did not perform many lumbar surgeries, so I was the only spine surgeon in town performing lumbar surgeries.

The second thing that was very good was that I had a good grip on how my patients were doing. This is an amazing opportunity for learning the practice of spine surgery. I believe that learning how to do a complex surgery is only half—or maybe less than half—of the equation in spine surgery practice. Most of the experience should come from what works and what does not. That is something that you cannot get in a large city practice. I can tell you with confidence that practicing in a small town was essential in the development of my skills and my understanding of the basics of spine surgery.

Because I was the only spine surgeon in town, I was followed by the local chiropractors. A few years into my practice, I asked myself as an open-minded person why I would question the work of chiropractors. I could not come up with a good reason, so I started befriending them. They came to my office and did presentations, and what they said and showed me made sense. They explained that when a patient experiences pain in their back, it means there is inflammation somewhere in their back, and I agree with that. They also explained that once you have inflammation, it leads to scar tissue and contractures, which I also agree with. It's a vicious cycle of inflammation, contractures, and more pressure. They explained that one of the reasons that pain becomes chronic is that pressure builds up in the tissue, and I agreed with that as well. They showed me a few techniques they performed to stretch the ligaments and decompress the joints, including the facet joints and the ligaments around the disc. By stretching the ligaments, they lowered the pressure in the tissue and gave the body the chance to decrease the inflammation. It sounded great so far.

It was not very long before I lifted a heavy object in my office and ended up with significant lower back pain. I was kind of waiting for this moment. I called up the chiropractor that I was most familiar with, and he fit me into his schedule right away. I was having significant pain in the right side of my lower back. I went to him, and he adjusted my back. I walked out of that office with minimal discomfort. I remember sitting in my car thinking I was a fool because I had written off chiropractors, and I was a little mad at myself for this. I usually solved a problem by looking at it from a different perspective, but I had violated my own rule.

From that point on, my practice was very different. I started working closely with chiropractors. I could now see the excellent work that chiropractors do because I sent my patients to them, and they were coming back to my office very happy.

Of course, I must point out that chiropractic care is not a silver bullet. In the world of spine care, there is no silver bullet because everyone is so different. If nonoperative care, including adjustments and injections, worked every time, my field as a spine surgeon would not exist.

I am not an expert in the chiropractic field. However, I will say that I receive referrals from chiropractors, and I send patients to chiropractors when I think it is an appropriate mode of treatment for them. I see chiropractic care as a way of adjusting the spine. I would describe it as high-amplitude, low-displacement adjustment of the spine. The purpose is to break up the scar tissue, stretch the ligaments, and eventually decompress the area causing the pain.

I was at a surgical conference once, and the surgeon who was giving the lecture did not seem familiar with chiropractic care. He was asked how many chiropractic manipulations would be reasonable before switching to another modality, and he said at most two manipulations. I did not have a question, but I raised my hand to make a point. I told the audience that I wanted to defend chiropractors as I had good knowledge of chiropractic care. In my experience, two adjustments would not be a reasonable number. I told them that it takes time and multiple adjustments for this modality to help. Some conditions might be better with fewer adjustments; everyone is different. For example, my wife pulled a muscle in her leg and went to a chiropractor. In her case, she needed only one adjustment. It's crazy. She complained about her leg for three months, then after one visit, I never heard her complain again.

Sometimes patients are in an inflammatory stage, and they are hurting quite a bit. This is when the injury has either just happened or it has been aggravated. At this stage, a patient cannot get manipulated at all because it just hurts. This stage can last a couple of months. Some people respond to one adjustment, some people do not respond at all, and some patients respond to treatment but the pain can come back once treatment stops.

Is chiropractic care a panacea? Of course not, but I often advise people to try it because it is a noninvasive approach that frequently pays dividends. If it works, it can save massive amounts of pain, money, and recovery time.

I am frequently asked whether chiropractic care or surgery works better. I constantly have to defend chiropractors to my surgeon friends, and I have to defend surgery to my chiropractor friends because chiropractors think surgery does not work.

Chiropractors and surgeons work on a different spectrum of the disease process. When a disease is mild, surgeons do not have anything to offer patients. This is when chiropractic care is invaluable. When chiropractic care stops working, then surgery could be an option. As healthcare providers, we should always realize it is not about who is right, and it is not about ego. It is about helping patients. That should be our primary goal.

Physical Therapy

As an orthopedic surgeon, I have significant experience with physical therapy, most of which I got in the first couple of years of my practice. When I started as an orthopedic surgeon, I performed general orthopedic procedures as well. I did hip replacements and knee replacements during the first couple of years of my practice. I loved trauma—for example, broken bones—so I continued treating trauma patients up until recently. Physical therapy is quintessential for a good outcome in that type of practice. As I mentioned in the previous section, this is my personal experience, and every patient is different. Therefore, I caution people about drawing conclusions based on what I am going to say.

I see physical therapy as a treatment that addresses the active and passive joint range of motion for strengthening and conditioning of muscles. This is essential in the extremities both before and especially after surgery. After hip or knee replacement, it is prudent to get the range of motion back. In the case of fractures, it is prudent to restore as much function as possible, which can only be done with aggressive physical therapy.

However, I have a different view about physical therapy when it comes to the spine. When it comes to spine surgery, most of the time, the culprit is deep structures such as the discs, the ligaments that hold the discs together, and the facet joints. It is very hard for me to imagine that physical therapy can stretch these ligaments efficiently. To stretch the ligaments around the injured disc or injured facet joints, the patient must get into an extreme range of motion. In these situations, it is very hard for a patient to tolerate these types of maneuvers. I believe chiropractic adjustments have the upper hand to loosen and decompress the deep ligaments and tendons.

My modality of choice preoperatively is chiropractic care. To mobilize the muscles, break up the scar tissue, and recondition the patient postoperatively, I like physical therapy. Admittedly, that is a very broad statement, but I genuinely believe chiropractic care is underutilized in spine care.

It is not just about being open-minded about other specialties. We should be open-minded within the specialty of spine surgery about new surgeries and procedures that become available. When a new surgery becomes available, we cannot be dismissive and hold on to old ways. Our patients deserve better. Tom Brady, the football quarterback, once said, "I think you can just go out and try to be the best you can be, deal with people with respect, with honesty, with integrity, have a high moral standard." That is how we should be as surgeons. Once a surgeon settles into a practice, they can develop habits, and it can be hard to learn new techniques. However, we owe it to our patients. We should always look at alternatives critically and evaluate them thoroughly, but we cannot be dismissive of new surgeries or alternative treatments just because they are inconvenient to us.

PART II: THERAPEUTIC PAIN PROCEDURES

When I decided to write this book, I had a very clear idea of what my message was going to be: to expose instrument companies and let people know that some instrument companies have successfully steered the science of spine surgery right into their pockets. However, once I started the actual writing, my goal went from just explaining this topic to producing an easy-to-read, helpful book that that brings patients my surgeon's point of view and twenty years of experience. Once they know this, I believe they will understand what a difficult task we face.

Each chapter has had its challenges, but this chapter about nonoperative procedures has been the most difficult. I have written this chapter at least five times and changed everything. I have changed this chapter from a very detailed and lengthy description of the procedures to a very brief description of the procedures without discussing the intricate details. I ended up settling somewhere in between.

It was challenging to write this chapter for two reasons. First, we do not understand precisely how pain starts; therefore, we do not have a targeted way of coming up with new techniques. Second, and more importantly, there is no definition of what a successful procedure means. Success could be anything from the pain completely going away after just one procedure to the other side of the spectrum with a patient getting just a minimal amount of relief.

The definition of success to me, which is absolutely a personal point, is if a patient gets a certain procedure and it causes enough reduction in pain for them to be happy and gain functional improvement. The other important point for me is that the procedure needs to achieve this without significant future costs or significant possible side effects. When I review the literature and the studies that have been done, I get the sense that success overall, as accepted in the world of spine surgery, is a complete resolution of the pain with one procedure only. That seems simplistic and unrealistic, but I understand how seductive that definition of success can be. Who wouldn't want that?

But before we talk about the treatment of pain, let's try to understand what pain is. Pain is a sensation in response to an injury. Of course, injuries can vary in severity, so the response of the body to any injury could be different in terms of magnitude.

The way the body responds to an injury is by stimulating hormones that lead to inflammation. Typically, people have a very negative perception of inflammation. When an area hurts, and the doctor says there is inflammation, the first thing you want to do is get rid of it. You take anti-inflammatory medication to eliminate the inflammation. However, inflammation is the body's mechanism for repairing the damage.

Think of inflammation as a construction site. You must place a fence around a construction site so nobody can enter and destroy your work. If people are walking around the site and things are happening, you cannot do your job. Pain is almost like a fence that is placed around a construction site. The pain creates a sensation that decreases the body's motion. That is the first thing that needs to happen so that repair can take place and prevent further damage. If you view it this way, pain is not a bad thing. It is a horrible sensation sometimes, but it is necessary for our survival. So is inflammation. Without inflammation, there is no healing.

We understand some of the pathways of pain. Material gets excreted and triggers the cascade of events leading to inflammation and pain. However, we do not fully understand the complete mechanism in the spine and in the intervertebral discs. We do know that when you have back pain or neck pain, it is caused by a cascade that has led to inflammation. There is strong evidence that points in that direction.

The first thing most doctors do, besides physical therapy, is to inject cortisone into the area, which is an anti-inflammatory. A lot of times, this works. When a patient asks if a steroid injection will mask the injury, my answer is that steroid injections are like a fire retardant. You have pain because your back is on fire, and we are putting out that fire. Cortisone does not heal the disc or heal the area. The goal is to lower or eliminate the pain, and that is what the injection is for.

The second powerful notion for pain being inflammation-related is that a lot of times, there is a delay between what the patient does and the appearance or worsening of the pain. For example, a patient might lift a heavy weight or get into a car accident, and he will not experience severe pain, or maybe even any pain at all, for days after the event. In addition, when you inject steroids, it takes two or more days for them to kick in and work. This is a very good indication that a cascade of inflammatory processes is responsible for pain.

For the first ten years of my practice, it was challenging to understand what was going on. Initially, I could not understand the pain behavior in my patients. A patient would tell me that they did not start having pain until two to three days after their car accident or two to three days after they fell. My initial reaction was disbelief. I doubted my patients. It was hard for me to understand that a patient would be pain-free or only experience a minimal amount of pain for a few days and then start experiencing severe pain. I even felt the patient might have talked to a friend who instructed them to fabricate the story for self-reward.

I had patients come to my office and say the pain just started out of the blue. Patients went to sleep with no problem and woke up with severe pain. I have had patients that had severe lower back pain and leg pain after sneezing. One patient was telling me that all he did was put his socks on. He got up one morning and took a shower to get ready for work. When he crossed his leg to put his socks on, he felt severe pain in the back going down his leg. He said it felt almost like he got stabbed in the back. I was baffled. How was it possible for a sneeze to rupture a disc? How was it possible for a patient to wake up with pain? And how was it possible that putting socks on could injure a person? Things only became clear about a decade into my practice, when I had my own experience with back pain. I was single at that time, and I drove to San Francisco on Fridays to meet my friends and have some fun. One weekend, I drove to Berkeley on a Friday afternoon, visited my mother and my friends Friday and Saturday, and returned home Sunday morning. When I got home, all I did was unbuckle my seatbelt with a minimal twist, and I had a sudden pain in my lower back that radiated down both legs. I was in severe pain for about five days, then the pain went away completely. What was going on? I was bewildered.

In my mind, I was a successful spine surgeon who was helping people; some of my patients had told me that I had changed their lives. At the same time, I had no clue what had happened to me and what was going on. I started analyzing my activities going back a few days. When I went to San Francisco to visit my friends, I went out and had a nice dinner and drinks on both nights. Then I remembered that I was at the gym on Thursday night (three nights before the onset of the severe pain). I remembered doing squats. I had become very comfortable with the weight I used for my usual workout. Therefore, on that night, I wanted to change things, so I added another ten pounds to my routine. I was more worried about my knees, so I wrapped my knees and was very careful with my form. I do not remember the weight I used, but I think it was around 260 pounds, so I had gone from 240 pounds to 260 pounds.

I could not believe that could be responsible for the onset of my pain three days later. I had been very careful with my posture. I felt I needed to investigate that. I went back to the gym and performed the same exercise with the extra twenty pounds plus another ten pounds, squatting a total of 270 pounds that day. I waited. I felt no pain on the first or second day. On the third day, I felt a twinge, and that twinge turned into full-blown pain. It appeared there was a delay in the appearance of pain after the initial insult.

I started experimenting more with my own back, and each time I performed squatting with the extra weight, the pain was triggered three days later. This was almost like winning the lottery. I was happy to discover something important from my own body. Everything began falling into place. When patients told me that it took them a few days to develop pain after an accident, I understood exactly how things worked sometimes, and I did not question them. If someone told me they woke from sleep with pain, I could advise them to think about two, three, or four days back to remember if they lifted something or did some strenuous work.

After I had performed surgery on a seventy-five-year-old male, he did very well for about three months, but then he presented to my office with increased pain. He told me he had no idea what happened, but he just started hurting one day, even though he had been doing well. I asked him to go back two or three days before he experienced the pain and to try to remember any activity that may have been excessive or more than his usual activity. He remembered that two days before the pain, he drove to Fresno to visit family, and that was a three-and-a-half-hour car ride. He stated that they went for a long walk once they got there. I felt that he must have tweaked his back during that trip. His pain returned to its baseline after a few days.

Things had become clear to me, and I could answer a lot of questions now. I highly doubted that coughing or sneezing caused rupture of a disc, as it is a physiological reflex. If the back is so weak that a disc could rupture from a significant cough or sneeze, then the emergency room would be stacked with back injuries during the wintertime. That does not happen. Therefore, the most likely explanation is that the patient does something, such as lifting an object or falling down, and is fine until something very trivial like a sneeze or reaching for an item ignites the inflammation a few days later.

I asked patients about their increased pain in detail, and each time there was an event going back several days that could explain it. Because there was a two-to-three-day delay, the patient did not initially correlate the pain with the earlier activity. I advise my patients that there is only so much we can do as health care providers, either doing injections or therapy. We see our patients about once a month; chiropractors see patients two to three times a week for thirty minutes at a time. But the patient is the one that spends the most time with their back, and they must lug around that back all the time. As health care professionals, what we can do for them is only a tiny part of what their back needs. The main part must come from the patient, and that is basically how they treat their back. This mostly means not lifting heavy weight as much as possible.

I often tell patients that before considering surgery, they should try a new career. I have patients who are in the landscaping business, so I start asking about their profession and how they run their business. Some have a small business, and they must perform the work themselves. I advise those patients to hire a younger person and pay them well to do the lifting. They tell me that they cannot afford an extra person. I tell them that the money they pay the young person to do the lifting is the best money spent. That money will ensure that the patient can work for a longer period with a much longer career. They will lose everything if their back goes out.

My experience over my twenty years of practice has taught me how to explain back pain, particularly chronic pain. When it comes to chronic conditions, I explain that the back has a limit. If a person stays below that limit, they will be fine and will not have back pain. However, if they do an activity that exceeds that limit, such as helping friends move or lift a couch, they start having pain. It is left for my patient to find that limit with trial and error and to stay on the safe side of that limit. That way, they can manage their pain. They need to have a memory chip in their head. If they start hurting, they need to recall what caused the increase in pain. They can compile enough data to tell them what their limit is.

The problem is that the limit can move over time, and a smaller weight can trigger the pain. Most of the time, the limit starts moving toward what I believe is the stress of daily activity. Throughout our day, we are constantly putting our backs to work. We do activities such as taking out the trash, going shopping, and getting bottled water. Even if your job is not strenuous, you are still constantly stressing your back through daily living. I would say that twenty to forty pounds is an average weight to lift in our daily lives, maybe an average-size suitcase. Let's say that a patient's limit that would trigger back pain is fifty pounds or more; then pain can be managed by activity modification. However, if this limit starts moving into the range of daily activity because of an accident and becomes thirty pounds or, twenty pounds, then the limit of the back is in the daily activity area. Once this happens, the pain becomes constant and can become very difficult to avoid. As the limit of the back moves toward daily activity and becomes less and less, these people eventually need surgical intervention.

The biggest question I get from almost every patient that comes to see me, is how they can move that limit above daily activity stress—in other words, how they can get better. Unfortunately, I do not have a good answer currently. It would be Nobel Prize-worthy research to find that answer. It seems that an injured disc in the lower back has a mind of its own. It might stay within the same limit for many years or, more likely, decrease toward daily activity limits.

As I have mentioned throughout this book, I like chiropractic manipulations and care. However, there is one area where I diverge from the chiropractors. When back pain and what can be done to improve back conditions are discussed, chiropractors unanimously say that you must strengthen your core. That means you do exercises to strengthen the muscles around the spine so that the spine can get stronger. That sounds great, and I agree that patients should exercise and strengthen their core. Why? Because it is not just one element. When you exercise to strengthen your core, you also eat right, lose weight, become healthier, and feel better about yourself.

However, I tell my chiropractor friends that muscle does not hold weight. You can build a tremendous amount of muscle around the core and the spine. However, when you lift a heavy weight, the force of that entire weight goes through the injured disc. No structure around the spine shares the load-bearing function of the disc. Even the facet joints in the lumbar spine are vertically oriented, and they do not bear the weight and share the load-bearing function. That means nothing can be substituted for not lifting heavy weight. The disc that is injured between the two vertebrae has a mind of its own, besides a new trauma. We do not understand why it goes in a certain direction, and we do not have the technology to alter that path.

I always tell my patients that they should exercise, lose weight, and strengthen their core. Exercise is prudent. But it's not everything.

Nonoperative Procedures for Neck and Lower Back Pain

This section will discuss the commonly performed nonoperative procedures for neck and lower back pain, but this will not be a complete list.

The procedures I will describe are the ones most recommended after chiropractic care when surgery hasn't been performed. In other words, these procedures are often suggested to people who have not improved with physical rehab, including physical therapy, chiropractic care, massage, acupuncture, and yoga. If the nonoperative procedures fail to give a patient reasonable pain control, surgery would be the next and last option.

Medications

I want to discuss medications briefly. This is a complex and controversial topic to discuss, and I went back and forth about whether to include it in my book. I do not want it to take away from my main message or draw unnecessary attention. However, I wanted to give the reader some sort of idea of what available medications can do.

To be clear: There is no medicine that I have ever used that I have liked in terms of treating pain in the neck, lower back, arm, or leg. Each time I have had relative success with a medicine, it has been followed by a complete failure.

The first type of medication that comes to my mind is narcotic pain medication, mostly because they are in the news so often. The whole world knows what these medications are and what they can do. I think narcotics are probably the only medicine we have that can help the patient to a reasonable degree, although they are not very effective for neuropathic pain, or pain related to inflammation. The other problem is, of course, that these can be habit-forming, and their efficacy decreases significantly within a short time. These medicines, including popular pain medicines like Norco, work well for only a few weeks before their efficacy decreases.

A patient needs to realize that pain is not just one entity. Different types of pain can coexist. At one end of the spectrum, there is a dull, achy pain that can be a burning sensation, and at the other end you have a pain that can be sharp and stabbing. Narcotic pain medicines are okay for controlling dull, achy, and continuous pain. In terms of sharp, stabbing pain, they are ineffective at best. I tell my patients if they have sharp, stabbing pain, they can take all the narcotics in the world until they are barely breathing, but they would still feel that pain.

There is one thing I have to mention. Due to the recent epidemic of narcotic addiction and narcotic overdose deaths, the government has come down hard on doctors about prescribing narcotics. I have heard of doctors' offices getting raided and doctors being arrested. This has made us very scared to prescribe minimal amounts of narcotics, even when a patient is in significant pain.

Currently, I only prescribe pain medicine such as Norco or Percocet for patients who have had surgery, and I do that only for about two months. From the beginning of the preop stage, I warn the patient that I will stop prescribing the narcotics after two months to prepare them. The bulk of the surgeries I perform are fusion surgeries. In terms of the lumbar spine, it takes four to six months for the fusion to solidify. The problem is that nonsteroidal anti-inflammatory medicines such as Motrin or Advil have been shown to decrease the rate of fusion, and this is detrimental to my surgery. I must juggle patients' needs for pain medicine with other aspects, such as losing my license to practice or going to jail.

Another pain medication group is called *nonsteroidal anti-inflammatories* (NSAIDs), and these are over the counter. These include Motrin, Advil, and ibuprofen, which are all the same medicine. I would throw Tylenol into the middle of that as well. These medicines are quite effective in terms of pain control, and there is a use for them. However, they are not even close to narcotic pain medicine when it comes to for pain relief.

I always tell my patients not to continue NSAIDs for an extended period. Every year or so, I read an article in a newspaper that a former athlete has developed significant kidney damage due to continued use of anti-inflammatories. During the first four years of my practice, I routinely placed patients on anti-inflammatories for two weeks, and I told them to continue for one month if it helped them. I advised them to stop after two weeks if it did not help them. After five years, I stopped that practice because I did not see any long-term benefit.

The third group of medicines is called *nerve-stabilizing drugs*, such as Neurontin. This group of medications is related to seizure medications. Their job is to stabilize the nerves. If a patient has arm pain or leg pain due to a pinched nerve, we can try these medicines. However, I have not seen any earth-shattering responses that would lead me to routinely recommend these to my patients. Muscle relaxants and antianxiety medicines are just for symptomatic control at best.

Nonsurgical Procedures

I divide the nonsurgical procedures into two categories. One category is injections that include glucocorticosteroid injections, the goal being to stop the pain by reducing inflammation. The second category is the procedures that are only for symptomatic relief. That means they help the pain, but they do not do anything to eradicate the source of the pain. The effects of this second group of procedures are temporary.

We know that pain starts with an inflammatory cascade. As I have discussed in previous chapters, there is strong evidence supporting that direction. Therefore, we would logically think that an injection of anti-inflammatories would be a solid therapeutic modality. I classify these injections, which include glucocorticosteroids, by how deeply they are injected.

The first category is an injection that goes into the muscle or soft tissue. These injections are generally referred to as *trigger-point injections*. The patient shows the doctor where the pain is located, and the doctor inserts a needle into the muscle of that area to inject a mixture of steroid and numbing medication so the patient can tolerate the procedure. Some doctors just inject numbing medication.

The next category would be procedures in which the needle goes down to the bone level. (This is a very broad simplification of different injections.) These injections include medial branch blocks and facet blocks. A facet injection uses an imaging machine, either ultrasound or X-rays, to guide a needle into the facet joint. There are different techniques and different opinions in terms of where the steroid should be injected. Some doctors believe the steroid needs to be injected into the middle of the joint. Other doctors think we should not place medicine in the middle of the cartilage because it could be corrosive; rather, it needs to be deposited around the capsule where most of the inflammation is present.

There is enough evidence in the research that shows the steroids could be deposited around the facet joint and not into it. That means whether a doctor injects the facet joint with steroids or injects the steroids around the joint, it works the same. With this recent information, doctors should avoid injecting the joint directly because that puts steroids onto the hyaline cartilage of the joint. This is like putting fine sand in the joint, because most of these medications are particulate in nature. Also, placing steroids around the joint could be done by ultrasound as opposed to X-rays, which means less radiation for the patient and doctor as well.

Next in the category of down-to-the-bone injections is the medial branch block. Again using imaging, the needle goes right outside the facet joint. This injection aims to calm the nerves that are going to the muscle and facet joints and hopefully decrease the back-pain causing muscle spasms. The indication for these two classes of injections are axial neck or lower back pain.

The last and third class of steroid injections to the spine is an injection under the bone and around the nerves into the spinal canal. These injections are called *epidural steroid injections*, and they could be performed either right through the middle between the two vertebrae or through the hole where the nerve exits the canal on the side. The idea is to put the needle closest to the areas that we think are the pain generators, which are the discs and the nerves.

We discussed that injections of corticosteroids differ in their depth—into the muscle or soft tissue, down to the bone, or under the bone and around the nerves and discs. The obvious question is which type of injection is the most efficient and therefore should be done first? Before answering that question, we need to go back and study corticosteroids.

The steroids that we inject to treat pain are a subgroup of corticosteroids called glucocorticoids, which are anti-inflammatory hormones produced in the suprarenal gland, also known as the adrenal gland, just at the top of the kidneys.

This group of hormones is not like some of the other medications we use. For example, we know exactly what a blood pressure medication will do once a certain dose is given to a patient. In terms of pain medication, a person knows how they feel if they take a whole pill or one-half pill. Unfortunately, steroids do not work like that. We truly do not understand precisely what is happening inside the patient. Sometimes they work, and other times they do not work. The same doctor can inject the same spot with the same steroid twice, and the patient might have two completely different experiences. The outcome with steroids is very unpredictable, at least in the spine.

One of the most frequently asked questions from my patients about steroid injections is, "What are the chances of it working for me?" I routinely tell my patients that these injections follow the rule of thirds. One-third of the time, it does not do anything at all. You come back and say, "I did not feel any difference besides the pain at the injection site." One-third of the time, it works. To what extent I cannot tell you, but it makes the patient happy in terms of pain relief. However, the symptoms eventually return. Then there is that last one-third group of patients that get long-lasting relief with these injections and even elimination of the pain.

Of course, I have not run research and crunched the data, but I see that the pattern, and the rule of thirds is about right. I tell my patients that the one-third of cases that have good, lasting relief and sometimes elimination of the pain is why we do these injections.

In my practice, I am quite involved in these non-operative procedures. Every two years, I go to conferences and get training for these procedures. I also perform them in medical facilities or my office. Therefore, I have good knowledge of what they are and what they do. I am mostly conservative about these injections. I often tell patients that if these injections worked every time, my profession as a surgeon would not exist. Who would have a complicated spine surgery if they could get better with just one shot?

Glucocorticosteroids are not benign medication. They are potent hormones, and we genuinely do not understand the long-term effects of the steroids. Research has shown that corticosteroids can weaken the bone quality if injected repeatedly, which could lead to significant fractures in the future. There are also reported cases of patients getting Cushing's syndrome with only one injection, but that is rare. Other possible adverse effects include hyperglycemia, increased appetite, weight gain, suppression of the immune system, and low serum testosterone.

There is another aspect of pain therapy that I dislike. Even though they do not involve an incision, these injections are still quite invasive for the body. When a patient has decided to get steroid injections repeatedly, besides weakening the bone, which is a major issue in itself, they can cause significant scar tissue inside the patient.

The spinal nerves are bathing in a sac filled with cerebrospinal fluid, called the *dura*. When I do laminectomies in patients that have received many epidurals, I encounter severe scarring around the dura and nerves. Yellow ligament gets stuck to the dura, making it very hard for me to dissect away the impinging structure and free the nerves. This leads to complications such as a dural tear that could lead to a dural leak and require repeated procedures. But the most important complication is an incomplete decompression of nerves, then an undesired outcome. The surgeon gets blamed for a bad result when the patient has inadvertently undermined their surgery by undergoing repeated pain-reduction procedures. This is mostly true for epidural injections.

It is easy to convince a patient who is in pain to undergo a procedure. However, doctors need to stick to ethics and always have the well-being of the patient in mind. A good example that comes to mind is laser surgery. Between 2008 and 2015, I was constantly seeing commercials for spine surgery on television. Commercials showed someone with back pain who would get surgery requiring only one Band-Aid. They showed a patient entering the facility with pain and agony and leaving the facility happy. The people who ran this facility were apparently spine surgeons. During that time, my patients constantly asked me if I performed the same kind of surgery or knew someone who did, or just asked me what I thought about it. My answer to those patients was that I am very active in research and development, I go to conferences twice a year, and I know people on the cutting edge of research. However, none of us knew what they were doing at that company. If it were a legitimate procedure, I would be out of business tomorrow. Who in their right mind would perform an extensive surgery with large incisions, screws, rods, and significant blood loss when the same effect could be achieved with just a needle and a Band-Aid? Also, I told them that if such a thing existed and was available, I would be the first to sign up and learn to do it, and I would offer it to my patients.

Guess what? There were significant news articles in 2019 that stated that the company was closed for good, and the chain was involved in multiple lawsuits. A judge awarded one plaintiff more than $200 million in damages. As I understand it, these people brought patients in and apparently promised to get rid of their pain. They required $50,000 in advance. They housed the patient in a very nice hotel right next to their facility. During the procedure, they injected a high dose of steroids, and the patient got relief from that. However, upon return of the symptoms, the company gave the patient a very standard response of sorry, but you were informed that the procedure might not work. The patients were then on their own and minus $50,000.

My message is that these pain procedures are not like pain medication that get cleaned from your body by the liver and kidney. Based on my interoperative observations, they caused permanent changes to the patient. I am not trying to say "Get the surgery." By no means. However, once a patient has decided to take the path of injections, then later decides to have surgery, they may have undesirable results, and the surgeon shouldn't be blamed for that. I genuinely believe having just a few procedures is safe. However, when you have too many, you may potentially burn your bridge to successful surgery.

The next question is where you start. As I said, this is very different from doctor to doctor based on their experience. There is no set rule in terms of the algorithm of treatment for a given condition. We know that overall, we follow the algorithm of physical rehab, injections, then surgery. But within the category of the injections, there are no set rules. I have personally explored the literature in detail. There is no indication of one injection being superior to other injections in terms of outcomes.

I have many patients who get better with a facet block for the neck or lower back. Some people do not improve, so I send them for an epidural injection, which works better for them. I also have many patients that have already had an epidural injection from a pain specialist, and they come to me for a surgical consultation. I then perform a facet block, and they get great relief from the facet block. I have many patients who have had significant relief with one injection, and they request a second injection when the pain comes back. My response is that we can proceed with that, but just because it worked the first time does not mean it will work again. The same is true for the other group. When I do one injection and do not get a favorable response, I tell them that a second injection might be completely different and could help quite a bit. However, if two injections of any type do not help a patient, I will abandon that treatment and move on to the next treatment. I can give you many stories about many patients with different situations and many different outcomes.

Likewise, the research is all over the place in terms of outcome. Research has not found a correlation between the dosage of the corticosteroid injected and the outcome. The fact that research cannot find that correlation tells me how unpredictable the outcomes of these corticosteroid injections are.

I will let you know my personal preference in terms of my practice. I do not want to create a controversy for no reason with what I am about to say. This is just a personal algorithm with no scientific basis. I do not have the data in terms of outcomes guiding me. Therefore, I select the procedures by their invasiveness. By following that rule, the order of the injections should be facet blocks, then transforaminal epidural injections to treat axial pain (neck or lower back.)

Suppose there is a component of arm or leg pain, and the patient has a pinched nerve. In that case, I immediately go to an epidural injection, which I believe is the better injection for radicular pain. For significant neck or lower back pain, I start with a facet block first. The facet block is a much less invasive procedure than an epidural injection. The facets are like knuckles when seen on the ultrasound. The target is big and not dangerous with this procedure. I have explained before that disc damage goes hand in hand with facet pain. If the facet block does not work, I will try an epidural injection.

I divide the risks of this procedure into two stratifications. One is procedure-based, and the other is gender-based. In terms of the procedure, a facet block is a very safe procedure with minimal side effects. As I said, the target is large and not dangerous. I still consider the epidural injection a very safe procedure. However, we are talking about much more sensitive structures such as the dura and spinal nerves. One of the common and known side effects of epidural injection is a spinal leak. If the needle goes slightly deeper than intended, the dura can potentially

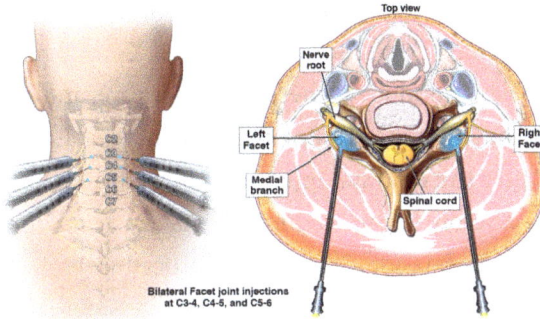

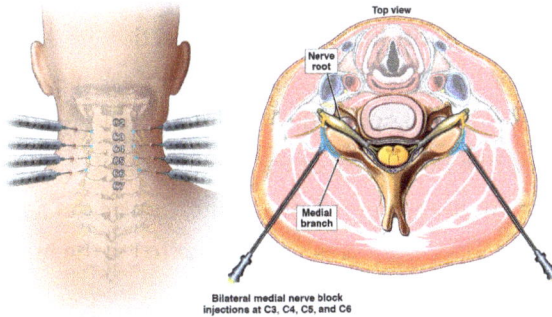

Figure 15: Cervical Spine Injections

be nicked, causing it to leak cerebrospinal fluid. If this leak is small, the patient will not have any problems. However, suppose the leak is larger, with the loss of a significant amount of cerebrospinal fluid. In that case, the brain floating in the skull starts settling, and the patient develops severe headaches.

The treatment for this condition, which is a dural leak, is either symptomatic relief with some pain medicine and muscle relaxants or, better, I would take the patient back to the operating room for a blood patch. That's where you take the patient's blood from the vein and inject that same blood into the epidural space where you think the hole is leaking the cerebrospinal fluid and patch it with blood that will clot. This is a very effective procedure, and it stops the symptoms most of the time.

The other complication of an epidural injection is nerve irritation. When you are doing this procedure using an X-ray, you cannot see the nerves. You have a good idea where the nerves are, and you try to avoid them, but the needle may irritate one of the nerves. I have patients that tell me that after the epidural injection, they have leg or arm pain that they never had before the procedure. This is not very common. Overall, an epidural injection is considered a safe procedure.

I can give you an example of how safe I consider it to be. My sister has a disc herniation at the level of C5-6. I performed a facet block on my sister, which did not help her. Through her primary care physician in San Jose, she was sent for an epidural injection in the cervical spine to be performed by a pain specialist. I did not ask her to find out who would be performing the procedure. I did not tell my sister to ask specific questions, like how many of these injections they have performed or to determine their credentials or qualifications. I did not ask her to let me find out who this doctor is. I just told her to get the injection and not to even worry about it.

The other level of complications is gender-based. This is basically due to the glucocorticoid medication itself. I seldom have a problem with men. Men might have some injection site pain, but that is about it. In women, these corticosteroids can affect their hormones, specifically before menopause. One of the problems is excessive bleeding during their menstrual cycles. This complication happens to about 25 percent of women between the ages of twenty-five and thirty-five, and they could bleed for about three to four weeks. This bleeding is mostly a nuisance and just involves some spotting the majority of the time. I have rarely had a patient that has bled a significant amount requiring a visit to their ob-gyn. There is not much that can be done to stop the bleeding. This only affects one cycle, and in their next cycle, they will go back to normal.

Many of my patients want to understand what is going on with their bodies. One question they ask is what these injections do. My analogy could be off, but this is the best I have come up with. I tell my patients that taking these injections could be the equivalent of taking fifty Motrin. You cannot take fifty Motrin because it will tear up your stomach; however, with the injection, the medicine is placed where it is supposed to go. These injections are just anti-inflammatories.

The next question is whether the injections repair disc damage. My answer is that the body does not have the capacity or capability to repair a disc; the force of gravity is too strong. For the body to have the chance of repairing an injured disc, the patient would need to be suspended in the air for an extended period, which is impossible on Earth. The only way to find out if the body can repair these discs would be to send the patient to the International Space Station for a month or two, then bring them back to Earth to see if their discs have been repaired or not. Running that experiment would be extremely difficult.

Another analogy I give to my patients with back pain is that their back is on fire somewhere, most likely their discs, and these steroids are like throwing fire retardant on it. The discs will not change, but hopefully the pain would go away. That is our basic goal. Once the pain goes away, we do not care what the discs look like.

I treat patients, not imaging studies such as MRIs. Sometimes a patient tells me that they have been told by their primary care provider that they have degenerative disc disease. They are quite afraid. I tell them that discs can wear out over time, just like any other part of the body. However, pain indicates whether there is a problem. If they have no pain, there is no problem. But if they are suffering from neck or back pain, then the damaged discs—as seen on an MRI—could be the source of their pain and they will need appropriate treatment to alleviate it.

I tell my patients that everything I do as a spine surgeon is to treat back and leg pain or neck and arm pain. Treating weakness and numbness are also goals, but my experience has been that when you treat pain, the numbness and weakness get better.

Patients want to know what they should expect and what will happen to them after a treatment. I tell them that it is almost like looking into a crystal ball. I have patients who have complete resolution of pain with one injection. With other patients, nothing that I try works, and I end up doing surgery on them.

I tell them that the very first steroid injection is the most important. If the patient does not respond to the first steroid injection, there is a likelihood that the patient will eventually need surgery. The patients who have a very good response to their first injection are the patients who generally do well and do not require surgical intervention. Therefore, I tell my patients that the first injection needs to be done right by somebody highly proficient and extremely qualified. As time goes on, a patient's problems could evolve, and therefore the response to steroid injections could change.

Procedures That Do Not Involve Steroid Injections

As I have explained, chronic neck or lower back pain is related to an inflammatory process. There is significant evidence for it. Therefore, injecting glucocorticoids (otherwise known as cortisone) addresses the root cause of pain and has the potential to eliminate it in its entirety. The procedures that I will review in this section try to intervene in the pathway of pain perception and do not address the cause of pain generation. These procedures, at best, give temporary relief.

Botox Injections

Botox is an enzyme that paralyzes muscle. It was first discovered in a bacterium called *Clostridium botulinum*. This enzyme interferes with the transmission between nerves and muscles and paralyzes the muscles. If you ingested this bacterium, you could end up dying because your respiratory muscles would become paralyzed and you would stop breathing. This is the same Botox used at cosmetic clinics to eliminate wrinkles.

As I mentioned earlier, a significant component of chronic pain in the neck or the lower back is muscle spasms. Botox injection is one of the armaments we have to treat neck and lower back pain, since it does nothing but paralyze the muscles. This can give us evidence of how much muscle spasms are contributing to severe neck and lower back pain. These procedures are done mainly pain management specialists.

For some reason, Botox is more effective in the cervical spine than in the lumbar spine. This is most likely due to the difference in the nature of the cervical spine and lumbar spine muscles, or it may have to do with the fact that the biomechanics of the cervical spine and the lumbar spine are entirely different.

Botox is a treatment modality that we can offer our patients, and sometimes it can be tremendously helpful to patients who have not found a treatment modality to help them. The downside is that Botox is not cheap, and it only lasts between four and six months. That means every four to six months, a patient must return to the pain specialist to receive Botox injections to get the relief they desire.

Radiofrequency Ablation

Radiofrequency ablation is a procedure in which the doctor uses a long probe, guided by an X-ray machine, on the outside of the facet joints at each level of the spine. The idea comes from anatomy. In spinal anatomy, the muscles in the back and facet joints are innervated by nerves coming from the spinal nerves. The spinal nerves come out through the neural foramina. Somewhere around the neural foramina, a branch of the nerve exits the main nerve, loops around the facet joint, and innervates the facet joints in that segment as well as the rest of the soft tissue in that segment. By placing probes right around the facet joints, these nerves are intercepted. Using radiofrequency, the very tip of the probe gets very hot. The whole idea is to cut the sensory nerves that supply the muscles of the neck and lower back, and the facet joints.

The good thing is that it can work, and it can help the patient quite a bit. The downside is that it does not get to the root of the problem. That means the pain will return. Radiofrequency ablation is a temporary procedure at best. In my practice, I have seen it last four to six months, if it works. Overall, radio frequency ablation is helpful for 15% to 20% of patients suffering from neck or back pain. I use radiofrequency ablation after a series of steroid injections because the goal is to eliminate the pain. However, as I have said, it is all individualized toward the patient.

Pain Pump

A pain pump is placed under the skin near the belly. The pump is around the size of a hockey puck or slightly larger, and it is connected with a tiny tube under the skin into a catheter that sits in the spinal canal right over the spinal cord. The patient must go to the doctor's office once a month to have the pump filled up with pain medication.

It works by delivering the medication right over the spinal cord in a very localized fashion. An analogy would be the irrigation of crops in the middle of the desert in Israel. Due to water scarcity, irrigation provides precious water right at the root to get the most out of the available water. The same concept applies here. The pain medication is delivered right into the nerves in the spinal cord. The medication does not have to travel through the mouth and digestive system before affecting the nervous system. This pump delivers a continuous preset amount of narcotic to the spinal cord, which the surgeon predetermines.

The biggest indication for this procedure would be a patient that is sixty-five years or older and has multilevel disc disease, which means more than three bad discs. Some people have deterioration of the entire lower back. In these situations, I truly believe that the benefits of an extensive surgery do not outweigh the risks. Instead of proceeding with a large surgery with an uncertain outcome, I would instead suggest that the patient tries the pump to see if that will provide comfort without sending them into a path of drug addiction. Just like anything else in the spine, every modality has a wide indication of usage. We could also think of the pain pump for a person with multiple surgeries without significant success or with continued residual pain.

Spinal Cord Stimulation

The technology of neurostimulators originates from pacemaker technology. For this treatment modality, a pain specialist inserts a probe over the spinal cord with an external battery for trial. If the trial is successful, the patient will go back to the operating room for permanent implantation. During this procedure, a surgeon opens a window into the spinal canal and inserts a long, thin electrode over the spinal cord. This electrode is connected through a wire that is tunneled under the skin and into a stimulator with a battery placed in the fat tissue. This stimulator is about the size of a pacemaker. The idea is to send electrical pulses to the spinal cord to disrupt the signals in the pain nerves and give the patient pain relief.

A spinal cord stimulator is a prime example of companies selling what I believe is questionable technology and being very successful at it. To invent a successful treatment modality, we have to have the science first; otherwise, it would be only a shot in the dark. In terms of the spinal cord simulator, in my opinion, the science is closer to science fiction. We do not know exactly where the pain pathways are in the spinal cord. However, we think the pain fibers between the lower body and the brain travel along the anterior, or front, part of the spinal cord. That is farthest away from the stimulator paddles. That means the electrical stimulus has to cross the entire spinal cord and disrupt only pain pathways without disturbing other signals. Such devices are mostly indicated for extremity pain. However, spine surgery is very successful in relieving leg pain; it is the back pain we need help with.

Analysis and Summary

It is challenging to sum up all the information we have so far and project into the future in terms of nonoperative procedures. One thing I would like my patients to realize is that we have come a long way. The science of spine surgery is as young as the invention of the MRI. Some surgeons might argue that we have been doing spinal surgeries for centuries, but I do not want to get into that argument. I prefer to say that spine surgery is a very young field with many unknowns. However, we have made good strides, and the future is very bright.

There would be no progress without thinking outside the box. I tried to study these injections for the first five years of my practice, and I eventually gave up because there were too many unknowns and questions. The questions were interconnected, which makes the answers even more difficult.

At this point in my practice, though, I am ready to give this another attempt. This time, I am armed with much more knowledge. I have seen more patients, and I have done additional research in the field of spine surgery. As I mentioned earlier, I have a special type of practice and I am heavily involved in research and development. I completely believe that I should not sit back and complain about the affairs in spine surgery if I am not doing anything to improve our field.

I do not want you to come away from the above discussion of nonoperative treatments for pain with any sort of feelings of despair or helplessness. Indeed, we do not yet have a cure-all, but better treatments are being developed all the time. Moreover, each person is unique, and what works for you might not work for a thousand others. Dealing with chronic pain is often a process of trial and error. The goal is to learn how to either cope with it, adjust to it, or take specific actions that will lessen or eliminate it.

In every case, the truth needs to be told, which is the only way things can improve. Patients deserve to understand the shortcomings of their doctors and the issues their doctors deal with. What makes matters worse is that some instrument companies, driven only by greed and through the use of consultants, will bring useless modalities to market. This derails the entire field and delays real progress. Every consultant needs to adhere to strict ethics and keep reminding themselves that they have a moral obligation to the well-being of their patients.

I tell my patients that the first thing I will teach them is that they must think that the glass is half full and not half empty, no matter what condition and what cross-section of life they are experiencing.

CHAPTER FOUR

~

Surgical Intervention

Spine surgery is a complex field of surgery requiring significant knowledge of biomechanics unique to the spine. A singular and vital structure of the spine is the intervertebral disc. I have explained the anatomy of the disc in detail in Chapter Two; however, it also has a complex function and motion.

There are two very different subspecialties in spine surgery. One is called *deformity surgery*, which is the treatment for scoliosis that was first developed at the turn of the 20th century. Its goal is to treat a deformed and twisted spine and bring it back to its normal alignment. In this field of spine surgery, diagnosis is easy, using long X-rays. However, the needed surgery could be very challenging, requiring long segments of fusion. In this subspecialty, the surgeon must decide whether surgery is indicated.

The second subspecialty comprises 90 percent of the spine surgeries that are performed. I call it "true spine surgery," and it is surgery performed for the treatment of pain. This is either axial pain (neck or lower back pain) or radicular pain (arm or leg pain). This surgery is performed primarily due to an injured disc, and it truly began with the invention of the MRI in the 1980s. The surgery itself is not as complicated as scoliosis surgery because it is performed in a localized area. However, the diagnosis remains an art form that surgeons learn through decades of practice. With this type of spine surgery, the decision to proceed is the patient's because they know how much pain they can tolerate.

It is absolutely crucial to recognize the significant difference between these two subspecialties. In scoliosis surgery, the surgeon is addressing what they see on X-rays and other imaging studies. In true spine surgery, the goal is to treat pain, and the surgeon focuses on the patient. In this case, everything that the patient does or says becomes a clue.

Scoliosis surgeons have the attitude that they can manage all spine conditions. After all, they do the most complex surgeries, and they are not shy about doing large surgeries; to them, it is routine. For the majority of spine surgeons who treat pain, it is all about the preservation of function. To summarize, scoliosis surgeons are more visual, relying on imaging of the patients' spines, and the rest of spine surgeons are more auditory, relying on what they hear from their patients.

A spine surgeon can follow two main principles and have a great career. The first principle is the ability to identify a pinched nerve on an MRI where the patient has extremity pain (arm or leg pain). Then he can go ahead and un-pinch the nerve, and that should relieve the extremity pain. The second principle is the ability to identify an injured disc when the patient suffers from neck or lower back pain. Then the surgeon can proceed with a fusion of the disc to relieve the neck or lower back pain. Spine surgeons can successfully treat 80 percent of patients using these two simple principles. To successfully treat the other 20 percent of patients, a surgeon needs to practice for decades and learn complex biomechanics.

During the first ten years of my career, I performed plenty of complex surgeries. For a stretch of about seven years, I did surgeries three and a half days per week and was still asking for more operating room time. I did very well in my practice. I had a good reputation and was not involved in any lawsuits, which is rare.

One important thing happens when you do so many spine surgeries. If you truly follow your patients over many years post surgery, you realize the significant limitations of spine surgery. Upon entering the second decade of my career, I started asking questions and viewing what we do in the world of spine surgery with a critical eye.

I always tell my patients that my job is not to promote surgery or talk them into surgery, because we cannot guarantee a perfect outcome. If they have concerns about the surgery or are afraid of it, I am obligated to answer all their questions and put them at ease. My job is to tell the patient if I can help them. If a patient has completed all the courses of nonoperative care and they continue with an amount of pain that is not acceptable for them, then the next step would be surgical intervention. *The patient* decides if they would like to proceed with that option, based on the risks and benefits explained by me.

Proceeding with spine surgery for a patient is a very difficult decision. Most of the time, a spine surgery involves fusing a number of vertebrae. This is a very slow process, and it could take up to six months to reasonably recover from surgery; in some cases, it takes up to nine months. That means not only does the patient need help through this process, but also they must have financial support and a favorable work situation that will allow them an extended absence. I have many patients that simply do not have the option. Many tell me that if they proceed with the surgery, they run the risk of losing their job and, most importantly, the health insurance for their family.

Each time I see a patient for an initial evaluation, I go over all the options, starting with nonoperative therapy and manipulative treatments. I then discuss the different stages of pain procedures and, in the end, I describe the surgery they would require if they continued to be symptomatic. Very frequently, at the first visit, as soon as I talk about surgery, the patient steps back and acts very apprehensive at my even mentioning surgery. I explain that I am not talking about the surgery to persuade them, but I just want to teach them about their condition. With some patients, I must tell them that even if they are in great pain, surgery would not be the best option for them. I explain that to them so they can understand that this leaves therapy and pain procedures as the only options available. That is something the patient needs to understand.

I am also frequently told by my patients that they have been advised by family and friends that if a surgeon starts talking about surgery, do not accept it because it will not help. It occurs less frequently that my patients tell me their friends and family have encouraged surgery because they did very well. My reaction to these situations is very standard. I explain to my patients that just like nobody's face is identical, everyone's back is different, and I cherish that because it makes my job very interesting.

Just because somebody tells my patient not to get surgery because they did not have a good experience, it does not mean my patient will not have a good experience with surgery. On the other hand, just because one person got better, my patient might not get better with surgery. What you hear from other people about back surgery does not matter because it is incredibly complex. Once a problem becomes very complicated, you must simplify it. I have a hard time seeing the faces of fear in my patients as I explain surgery. I tell my patients that the best thing is not to do surgery, but once it comes to the point that you cannot live with such pain, surgery becomes necessary.

There are instances in which I would like to talk a patient into surgery. These are the patients whose symptoms are not very severe but are also not very mild. These are the patients that could go on for a few years before the pain gets significant. However, over those few years, they will have a very low quality of life requiring significant pain management. With these patients, early intervention can equate to better results. I explain to my patients that I can un-pinch a nerve, and I can immobilize or remove a bad disc. However, if there is compression for an extended period with scar tissue inside the nerve, there is not much I can do for that as the brain can get used to receiving all these pain signals. In addition, if they have had pain for an extended period because of bad discs and they have lost muscle function and developed atrophy, the muscle weakness is not likely to get better. Therefore, the results of delayed surgery would not be as good as early intervention. I tell my patients if they have had the pain for one year and I do the surgery, I can bring the pain down to about zero or one. But if they have had the pain for five or six years, I can only get the pain down to about three or four. I often feel a dichotomist strategy on what to do with some patients.

My practice and ethics tell me that I cannot promote surgery, and it is the patient's decision. Sometimes I feel that I should encourage surgery by guiding the patient through their condition, but I do not do that. This can be something I struggle with. I had a patient with a moderate-sized disc herniation. She was a woman in her thirties with a large herniation at S1. The patient had an impingement of the nerve root causing significant leg pain. This is a rare situation, but it does happen. I tried to take my time to avoid surgery, and we tried different injections. About two months after my first visit with the patient, nothing was working, and she decided to proceed with surgical intervention.

When I did the surgery and opened the canal, I could not find the disc. I panicked for a minute and thought I had either done surgery at the wrong level, on the wrong side, or perhaps looked at the wrong patient's MRI. I am always very diligent and never take anything for granted. When I do surgeries, I have the patient's MRI in the operating room.

In this case, I could not find the disc herniation even though I thought I would be facing a huge disc. I became alarmed. I went up and down the canal and checked the X-rays and my consent form. Everything checked out. I was at the correct level and on the correct side with the correct patient, and I had the MRI right in front of me. But there was no herniation. I opened the canal, unroofed the canal, inspected all the neural structures, and they were all free of impingement.

I discovered that the extruded material in the canal was mainly the gelatinous material, which is very well hydrated. It had quickly dried up, and as it did, it pulled the nerve into the canal and caused scarring. Unfortunately, there is not much that can be done for these patients. Once the tissue scars around the nerve, it cannot be taken off the nerve. If you start manipulating the nerve, the patient will get severe and relentless pain called *complex regional pain syndrome*. Even touching the skin causes severe pain in these cases.

The point of this story is that I questioned whether I should have intervened earlier. I do not know whether it would have mattered with the condition that she had. These conditions are rare, but they do happen. There is something to be said about proceeding to surgical intervention sooner than later. To this day, my practice is mainly based on the patient deciding whether they want to proceed with surgery and the patient deciding on the timing of the surgery. That's one of the reasons why I have never been sued for any procedure I have ever done in twenty years, which is rare in the practice of spine surgery.

The MRI shown on the left in Figure 16 is of a twenty-six-year-old woman who came to see me with two months' history of severe lower back and leg pain. She had tried physical therapy but could not tolerate it because of the pain. An epidural steroid injection did not work for her, and she was clearly a surgical candidate for a lumbar laminectomy at L5-S1. Because she was so young, I wanted to avoid surgery. I had an intuition that we should wait, and so we did. I brought her back a month later and got a new MRI for reevaluation. The second MRI, Figure 16 on the left, showed that the majority of the disc problem had disappeared and there was no impingement of nerves. The patient also felt a lot better than she had a month earlier.

Both cases I have presented are very rare. My goal in presenting these is to explain how difficult the job of a spine surgeon is. Plenty of times, we have to rely on our intuition and experience to manage a condition,

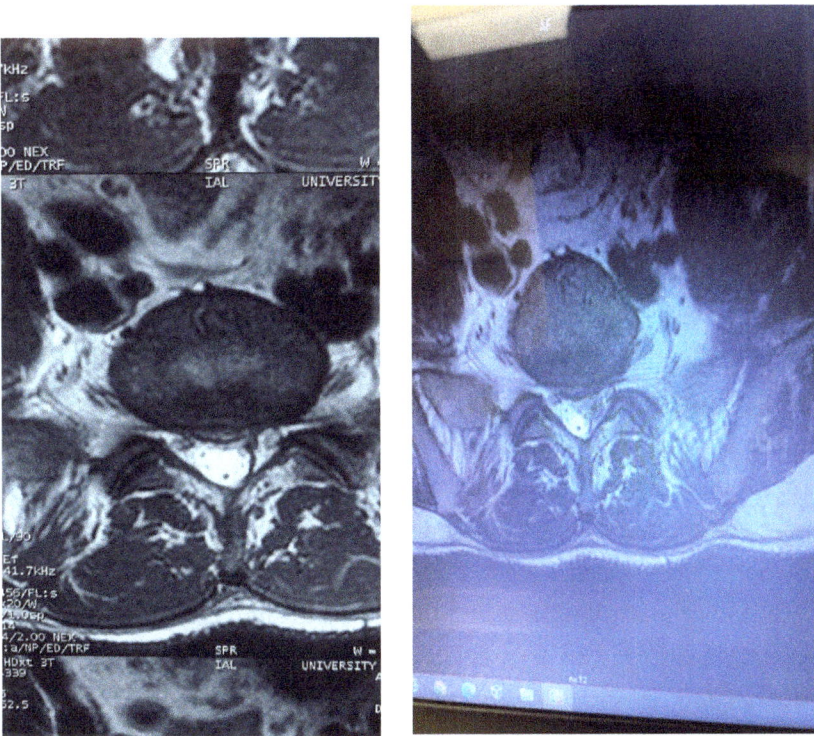

Figure 16: MRIs Taken Two Months Apart

and intuition requires decades to mature. It's not a skill taught in medical school.

Scoliosis

Scoliosis is a condition that causes significant malalignment in the spine and can lead to underdevelopment of the chest cavity and difficulty breathing, which has important health implications. But scoliosis is not considered a painful condition.

There are two main groups of scoliosis patients. The first group is adolescents. The prevalence of scoliosis in males and females is equal.

However, the risks of progression are much higher in young females, and they are the ones that mostly require surgical intervention to stop the progression of the curve. The worst time for progression of the scoliosis curve is when female adolescents start their rapid growth. At that time, young girls become susceptible to the curve increasing in magnitude.

When a patient is referred to a scoliosis surgeon, it is determined if the curve is very bad and needs to be fixed right away or if the curve is moderate and can be watched to see if it gets worse. If the curve is not growing very rapidly, they might try bracing.

Scoliosis surgery spans an extended region, and it can require screws and rods spanning five to eight or even more motion segments. The reason for doing the surgery is to visibly improve the curve and measurement of the spine through different techniques.

Sometimes when a young person has a mild curve, they can go decades without experiencing problems, but the curve can start progressing again due to uneven wear. Once that happens, many such patients end up with pain that can worsen. In that situation, the indication for surgery later in life is due to the pain, and the patient decides whether to proceed with the surgery. I will not go further into the surgical treatment of scoliosis in this book as it is not my area of specialty.

Radicular and Axial Pain

Most spine surgeries address one of two problems. One is when a herniated disc or bone spur is pinching a nerve. This results in pain in the distribution of that nerve, which we call *radicular pain*. This can be very debilitating. It is often performed when a patient does not respond to nonoperative care, so we must perform surgery to unroof the nerve. This hopefully will decompress it and relieve the symptoms by removing what is causing the impingement.

The other reason for surgery is to address a pain that is originating from an injured disc and causing neck or lower back pain. We call that *axial pain.* In this case, the disc causes arm or leg pain without pinching a nerve, and the nature of the pain is different. Just as I discussed earlier, we try nonoperative treatment first. This includes physical rehab, manipulations, and pain procedures, including steroid injections. If these do not work and the patient is suffering from debilitating neck or lower back pain, we must surgically address that injured disc.

In this situation, we usually go in from the front of the spine to remove as much of the disc as possible and replace it with a block spacer. This is what we call *fusion surgery.* Over the last ten years or so, another surgery has been introduced to address the injured disc, called *disc replacement surgery.* The goal is to remove the disc and place a prosthesis instead of fusing the two bones, which moves and maintains the motion in that segment. I will be discussing disc replacement at the end of the chapter.

This encompasses about 90 percent of the procedures we do for spine-generated pain. Of course, there are other surgeries. For example, if a vertebra is fractured or if there is a tumor or an infection, we must address those issues. In this book, I am discussing mainly the pain generators of the spine.

Laminectomy

Laminectomy is one of the most-performed surgeries in the world of spine surgery. *Laminectomy* means removal of the lamina.

The lamina is a flat bone covering the spinal canal where the spinal cord and the nerves traverse from the head down to the sacrum. This cortical bone is one of the strongest, densest bones in the body. It is like an arch, such as when you enter a garden. The concrete walkway is the back of the vertebral body. The two columns that support the top of the arch are the pedicles, and each side of the top is the lamina. If a bunch of arches are placed in a row, it forms a tunnel that is like the spinal canal. At each level, a nerve exits the canal. The nerves are named according to the bone where they exit.

Lumbar Laminectomy and Surgical Fusion (L4-5)

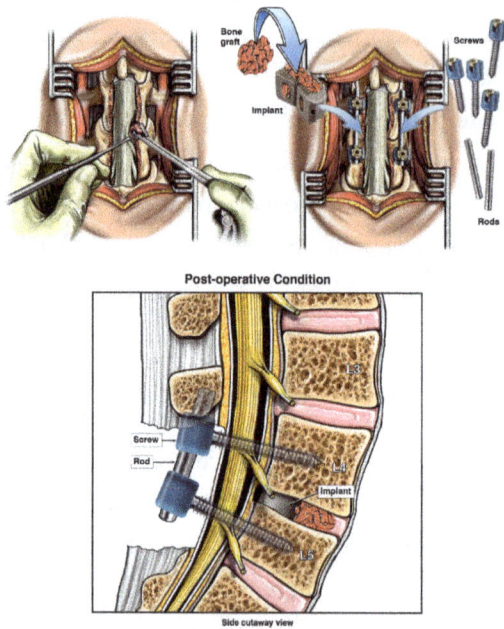

Figure 17: Lumbar Laminectomy and Surgical Fusion

Most of the time, a laminectomy is performed to decompress a pinched nerve. Compression of the nerve may be in different areas, depending on what is causing the impingement. The structures surrounding the spinal canal include the disc in the front, which traverses the entire width of the vertebral body. The facet joints are present on the corners, and they can hypertrophy and start encroaching on the spinal canal. The yellow ligament is in the very back and connects the two consecutive laminae to each other. It is called "the yellow ligament" because it looks yellow due to the dominance of a type of fiber called *elastin*. The elastin, as you might expect, makes this ligament very elastic.

I have covered disc herniation in another chapter. Once a herniation occurs, this can have different forms. It could be a localized bump, or it could be broad-based, spanning the width of the spinal canal. Multiple factors can cause this, and so it needs to be approached differently. The disc's job is to support the two vertebrae and support the weight of the body. The disc works like a shock absorber, as it contains a significant amount of very soft hydrophilic material in the middle. This is supported by a significant number of ligaments that wrap around the nucleus pulposus.

The disc is like a tire, but it contains gelatinous material instead of air. If there is an injury to that rim of connective tissue, the disc cannot perform its job of supporting the two bones very well. Depending on the size of this injury or damage to the fibrotic ring, the gelatinous material can start seeping out. The rate of the seepage depends on the size of the damage. The damage can be on a small molecular level, such as a crack, and it would take years for the disc to lose its function. If the damage is massive, it can start settling almost immediately or within months.

I stress to my patients that the real reason for symptoms is inflammation. Disc herniation can cause pain in two ways. First, the material in the center of the disc can cause chemical inflammation of the nerve, and second, herniation can produce mechanical compression of the nerve and cause numbness and weakness.

We usually perform a laminectomy under two circumstances. One is in a young person who has sustained an injury and has a disc herniation at a level of the spine to one side. Once the patient fails nonoperative care, we approach the surgery from the back. After determining the level, we will do surgery by scraping the muscle off the bone. If the surgery is minimally invasively, we insert and dilate the tube to have an area to do our surgery. Once that is done, part of the lamina is drilled out, mostly the inferior part. Then the yellow ligament between the two laminae is removed. This gives an access window to the spinal canal. In this situation, the dura—the sac that the nerves are traversing—is identified and pulled out of the way. Now we are looking straight into the herniated disc that is pinching the nerves.

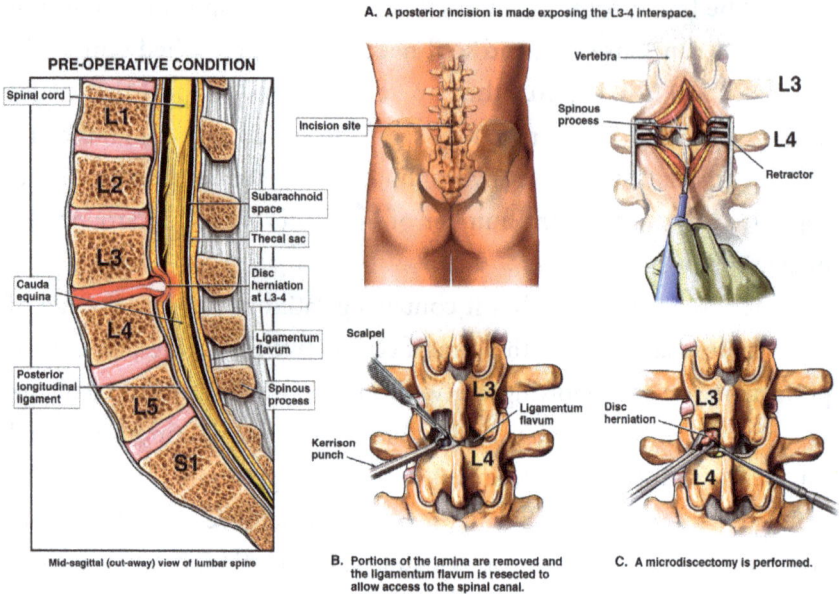

A. A posterior incision is made exposing the L3-4 interspace.

PRE-OPERATIVE CONDITION

Mid-sagittal (cut-away) view of lumbar spine

B. Portions of the lamina are removed and the ligamentum flavum is resected to allow access to the spinal canal.

C. A microdiscectomy is performed.

Figure 18: A Posterior Incision Is Made, Exposing the L3-4 Interspace

At this moment, we use a knife or laser to cut only the part of the disc that is extruding into the canal. Often this comes out as one piece, though it could be multiple pieces. A good surgeon must make sure all the material extruded into the canal is removed. If a ligament or a piece of the extruded disc is left behind, the patient might not have pain relief, and the surgery would fail.

The second reason we do laminectomies is in the older population. In this population, because of ongoing wear and tear and disc settling, a phenomenon called *spinal stenosis* occurs. Most of the time, this is circumferential. That means that the disc, facet joints, and yellow ligament all contribute to this stenosis. In this situation, we must remove the laminae on both sides, widen the canal, and probably remove part of the facet joints to ensure all the nerves are decompressed.

This surgery could be followed by a fusion or could be done by itself, and that decision is made by the surgeon depending on the patient's symptoms. For example, if the surgeon thinks the patient's back pain is generated

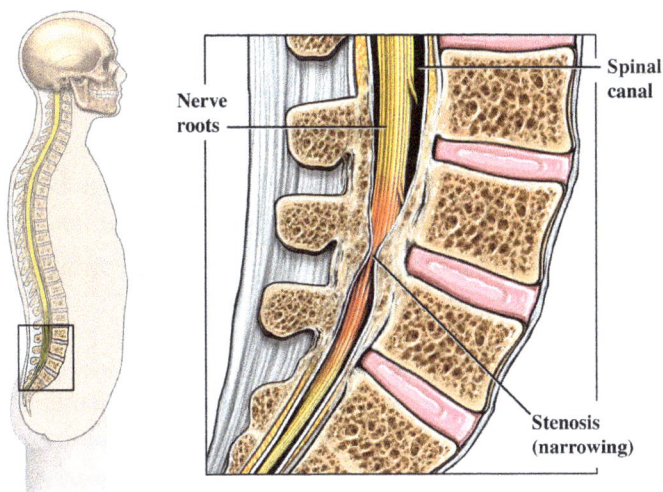

Figure 19: Spinal Stenosis

by the injured disc as well, the best treatment would be to decompress the nerve and fuse the level. The surgeon might determine that if the stenosis is too severe and a significant amount of bone is removed to accomplish the decompression, that would cause considerable instability, which obligates the surgeon to fuse the level to stabilize it. These are all decisions that are made by the surgeon, based on their training and experience.

I am incredibly passionate about laminectomy surgeries. It's upsetting to me that, I believe, spine surgeons do not currently understand the importance of the lamina. I have engaged in many conversations with my colleagues about this. I stress the importance of lamina and that we must save as much lamina as we can in any surgery. I would say that the entire world of spine surgery believes lamina is just a door to the canal, and we can just get rid of it without any consequence. Their analogy is that the lamina is like the top of a can. To get access to the contents of the can, the lid must be blown off. I have a very different view, and I find myself in arguments with other surgeons about this.

First, we need to understand the biomechanics of lamina. As I have mentioned in other parts of this book, when we first started doing fusions as orthopedic surgeons, we knew the value of the immobilization of two bones that are supposed to bond together. Initially, we used lamina as an anchor. The devices we had were sublaminar wire, cables, or hooks that hooked the lamina from above or below and connected to a rod.

The invention of pedicle screws changed everything. Once orthopedic spine surgeons decided that the pedicle screw was a better device to immobilize the spine (which I will later explain is wrong), the lamina became a nuisance. The lamina did not have any value to spine surgeons anymore; it was just a strong door that needed to be blown off or removed to perform spine surgery. The current thinking in spine surgery is to remove all the lamina and even go wider to ensure all the nerves are decompressed. There is no respect for the lamina in the world of spine surgery. We need to go back to try to study lamina.

Muscles attach to the spine through different processes: the spinous process and two transverse processes, the facet joints and laminae. They also attach to different levels in the spine. The transverse processes, spinous processes, and the other parts of the back of the spine converge on the lamina. That means the lamina is the primary connector that transfers all this muscle tension into the vertebral body to control the movement of the spine. It is very well known that the lamina is a solid cortical bone, and it blends with the inside wall of the pedicle, which in turn blends with the back side of the spinal vertebral body, which is the location of the most important force transmission. If you follow this logic, the lamina is almost like a handle for the spine.

There are two essential properties of the lamina that we need to understand. One is that the entire lamina is not very strong. The upper half is solid, but the lower half is not as strong. I would say that the upper half of the lamina is two to three times stronger than the lower half. I have not done studies to come up with this number, and this is purely my guesstimate.

The second most important thing is that I have never seen lamina causing a problem. Everything around the lamina causes issues, including the facet joints and the yellow ligament, but not the lamina itself. I always explain to my colleagues that it is prudent to save and maintain the upper half of the lamina during surgery. That is important because, throughout my years of doing complex surgery, I have learned that if you must remove the lamina, you can achieve anything you want to achieve by removing the lower half of the lamina only.

I have had to remove the upper half of the lamina only a few times in my entire career. One time, the disc traveled down behind the vertebral body below the disc level. In this situation, I wanted to make sure that I removed all the disc material; therefore, I had to remove some of the top part of the lamina of the vertebra below and inspect the neural structures. However, I remember that I only had to perform this kind of inspection a few times. At that point in my practice, I did not have my current knowledge.

In later chapters, I will explain how the evidence shows that a pedicle screw is a terrible way of immobilizing the spine. In short, I will tell you here that the pedicle screw is inserted in the vertebra and uses cancellous spongy bone for its anchor. This spongy bone is fragile. I believe that any successful device developed in the future would take advantage of the lamina for immobilization of the spine. As I mentioned above, I believe the lamina is like a handle for the spine. When talking to my colleagues, the analogy I use is that you lift a suitcase by its handle; you would not shish kabob a suitcase. Of course, my argument has fallen on deaf ears so far. The notion that the pedicle screw might be suboptimal in fixation of the spine is almost blasphemous in spine surgery. Unfortunately, we learn in orthopedic surgery that the solution to any problem is a screw.

It is important to save as much lamina as we can with every patient. At this point, we might not have a device available for laminar fixation, but I have no doubt that it is in our future. I tell my colleagues that we need to save as much lamina as possible because if the patient requires surgical intervention in the future, we will be able to use those devices. Once all the lamina is taken out, unfortunately, the patient might not be a candidate for new technology down the road. I would like to stress to my colleagues to be more courteous to the lamina and only remove the part necessary to get the work done. I'll say again: It is important to try to preserve as much lamina as possible. I hope my colleagues hear that message.

Fusion

Fusion is a surgery performed to form a bone bridge between two vertebrae so they become one bone. The idea is that if the disc between the two vertebrae is injured and causing pain, by fusing the two vertebrae we eliminate motion and therefore eliminate pain.

To truly understand this surgery, we need to go back to its origins. I should reiterate how we got here in this section. The technique of spinal fusion all started from the treatment of scoliosis.

In the mid-1950s, Dr. Paul Harrington from Baylor College of Medicine in Houston, Texas, introduced Harrington rods. Dr. Harrington used a rod and two hooks to spread apart a curved section of the spine to straighten it. We did not get a perfect correction of scoliosis in this manner, but that was the beginning.

After that, Dr. Eduardo Luque from Mexico City came up with a new technique. He put rods on each side of the spine over the lamina, threaded wires underneath the lamina, and twisted the wires over the rods. The spine slowly conformed to the straight rods, which was a good way of correcting scoliosis curvature. Until this time, patients had to wear a brace, but Dr. Luque's technique made braces obsolete. We treated spinal deformity with fusions from the mid-20th century until the 1970s and 1980s.

At the beginning of the 1980s, MRIs became available. You can argue the field of spine surgery began at that point; before the MRI, we had nothing. There was no way of looking at a disc and determining if it was injured. When the MRI became available, we were able to identify the source of back pain. It was natural to think about eliminating the disc as a pain generator and treating it with fusion. We already had experience with the fusion from scoliosis deformity surgery, and we applied the same principles to spine surgery.

When we started doing these surgeries, the bulk of spine surgeons did not use any instrumentation, screws, or hooks. They would place a bone graft between the two vertebrae and hope the graft would turn into a solid bone. This required bracing after the surgery. Overall, the surgery was not very successful, because there was a significant amount of non-union. The fusion rate was about 75 percent, which was not very good odds for healing for a surgical outcome. Therefore, orthopedic surgeons started looking for devices to immobilize the spine. They investigated whatever was available from scoliosis surgery. First, they tried sublaminar wires. Then they tried hooks. When the pedicle screw was invented, it became very popular because it was in line with orthopedic principles.

The surgery could be done without the screws, but the whole idea for using them was that by adding the screws, you would increase the fusion rate and avoid returning to the operating room for redo surgery. There was initially quite a bit of backlash from the government about using these pedicle screws because there was simply no evidence that they worked, and there were unsatisfactory results.

As a matter of fact, in the world of spine surgery, there was a dichotomist approach. Spine surgeons have either orthopedic training or neurosurgery training. Orthopedic surgeons do scoliosis treatment, and they are very familiar with screws and rods and basic carpentry; therefore, the use of screws became the preference for orthopedic spine surgeons. Not using screws became the preference for neurosurgeons performing spine surgeries. In the 1980s and 1990s, neuro-spine surgeons were very skeptical about the screws.

A paper was published in 1993 that indicated screws worked perfectly. Once that paper came out, it gave the instrument companies and surgeons the green light to use pedicle screws routinely. Medical device companies encouraged and promoted these screws with unfounded evidence. Eventually, neurosurgeons gave up their fight and started using the pedicle screws. By the year 2000, most fusion surgery was getting screws placed.

Here comes the twist. In the late 1990s and early 2000s, six independent, multicenter, prospective, randomized studies—some award-winning—came out and said that the screws *do not work*:

1) *Spine*, 1997 December 15; 22(24): 2813-22. 1997 Volvo Award winner in clinical studies. The effect of pedicle screw instrumentation on functional outcome and fusion rates in posterolateral lumbar spinal fusion: a prospective, randomized clinical study.

2) *Spine*, 1999 March 15; 24(6): 553-60. A randomized prospective study of posterolateral lumbar fusion: Outcomes with and without pedicle screw instrumentation.

3) *Spine*, 2002 June 1; 27(11): 1131-41. Chronic low back pain and fusion: a comparison of three surgical techniques: a prospective multicenter randomized study from the Swedish lumbar spine study group.

4) *Spine*, 2002 June 15; 27(12): 1269-77. Long-term functional outcome of pedicle screw instrumentation as a support for posterolateral spine fusion: randomized clinical study with a 5-year follow-up.

5) *Journal of Spinal Disorders & Techniques*, 2002 June; 15(3): 187-92. The influence of lumbar lordosis on spinal fusion and functional outcome after posterolateral spinal fusion with and without pedicle screw instrumentation.

6) *Medical Science Monitor*, 2003 July; 9 (7): CR324-327. Clinical outcome in monosegmental fusion of degenerative lumbar instabilities: instrumented versus non-instrumented.

The studies all concluded that the addition of screws posed a significant risk to the patient. The outcomes for patients who received the screws and those did not were absolutely the same. The most recent paper that looked at this specific topic, as of this writing, came out on December 1, 2018, in the journal *Spine*, and it came to the same conclusion.

Two decades have now gone by since the first of these published studies, and things still have not changed in the world of spine surgery. We keep ignoring the evidence and keep on truckin'. The evidence against the screws is overwhelming.

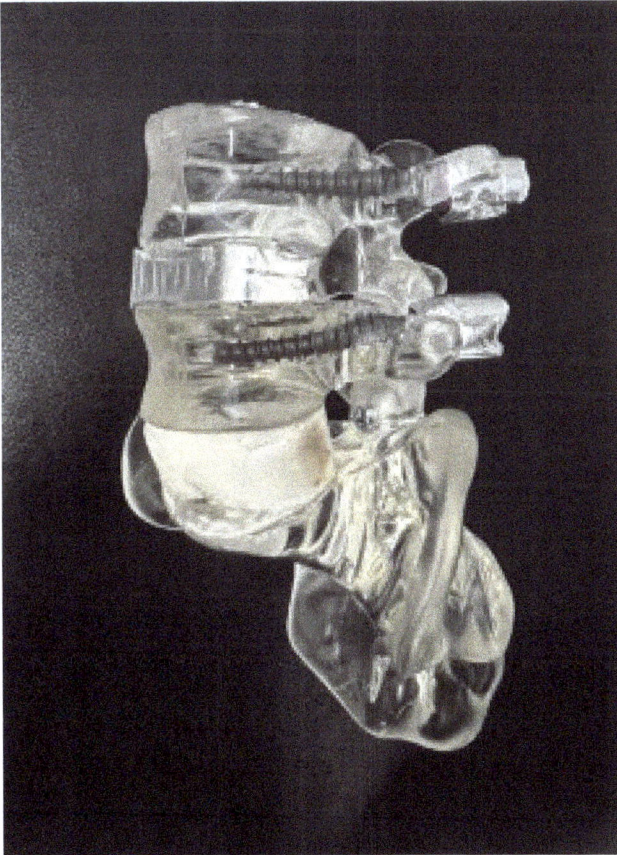

Figure 20: Pedicle Screws in Middle of Pedicle

Posterior Fusion

Whether to perform the fusion from the front only, from the back only, or from a combination of the front and back is a very complex decision that should be left to the surgeon performing the surgery, and most importantly, guided by the problem. The decision is based on the surgeon's training, experience, and understanding of the spine.

In the posterior fusion, posterior elements are utilized—the lamina, facet joints, and spinous processes—to create bone between the two vertebrae. In this surgery, an appropriately sized incision is made over the surgical area, and the muscle is divided. On each side of the spinous processes, the muscle is scraped off the bone, and retractors are inserted. The possible laminectomy and surgical decompression are performed. (See Figure 21 below.) The bone is decorticated to make it raw, and the bone graft is placed over the exposed bone.

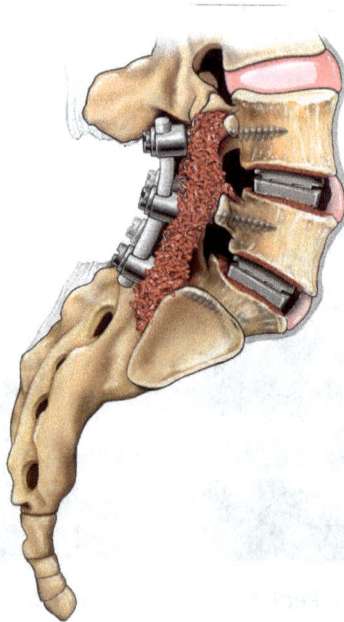

Figure 21: Pedicle Screws Inserted in the Vertebrae, Connected by a Rod

A decision must be made now. In an instrumented fusion, pedicle screws are inserted in the vertebrae above and below, then connected by a rod. That would be the end of the surgery. However, surgery performed without instrumentation is done after placing the bone grafts.

Anterior Fusion

In the anterior fusion, the spine is approached from the front. If it is in the cervical area, it is much easier. Once an incision is made in the skin, other structures are spread but not cut. The esophagus and trachea are spread medially, and the carotid sheet is spread laterally. The anterior cervical spine is exposed, and retractors are placed. Then the disc is taken out and scraped with different instruments. A spacer is placed, which could be cadaver bone, a piece of specialized plastic, or a titanium cage. This is packed with bone substitute and tamped into the disc space.

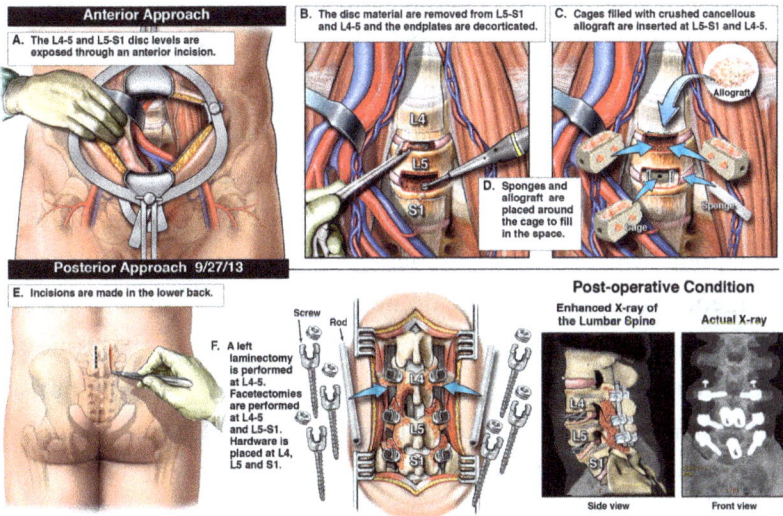

Figure 22: L 4-5 and L5-S1 Lumbar Spine Anterior and Posterior Surgeries

In the lumbar spine, dissection is a little more complicated. There are vital structures in front of the lumbar spine. I have an approach surgeon or abdominal surgeon make the approach for me. They get in there first by making an incision over the abdominal wall, going under the abdominal muscles, then sweeping the abdominal contents to one side. Once that happens, it is my turn. I repeat the procedure that I have described above for the cervical spine.

Different-sized scrapers are used to take out as much disc material as possible from the disc space. An appropriately sized spacer—again made from cadaver bone, a special type of plastic, or titanium cage—is packed with bone substitute and tamped into the disc space. That is an *anterior fusion*.

What is my preference? Doing an anterior fusion in the lumbar spine because it allows multiple options. The spacer can be inserted straight from the front (ALIF procedure), from the side (XLIF procedure), from the angled back (TLIF procedure), or from straight back (PLIF procedure). So, an anterior fusion in the lumbar spine can be done from four different angles. In the cervical spine, there is a straight front technique, and that is about it. A patient can go to different doctors, and each doctor could have a different preference. The question is why ten spine surgeons could have ten different ways of doing the same thing.

I have an answer for that. It might not be the most appropriate answer, but I will try my best. There is so much variety from surgeon to surgeon, purely because we do not understand biomechanics well. There has been significant research to try to address this issue and which technique is better. The problem I see is that we are not using biomechanics that are specific to the spine. When I go to a conference, there is no mention of biomechanics. In Chapter Eight, "The Future of Spine Surgery," I will explain the true biomechanics of the spine in detail. I have spent the past five years of my practice developing these principles.

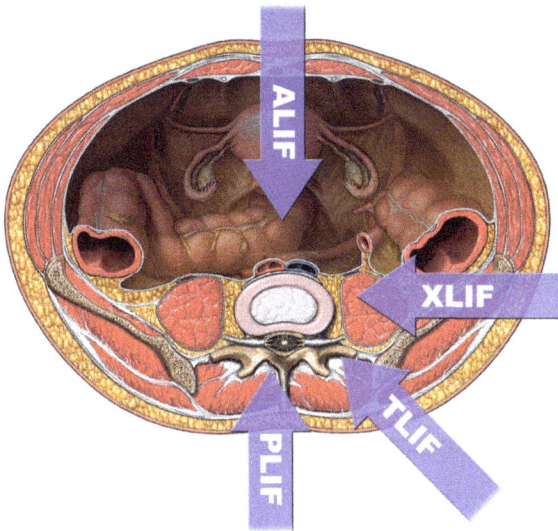

Figure 23: Four Different Angles of Lumbar Spine Anterior Fusion

The spine is a mechanical device. The laws of physics govern it. However, none of that is taken into consideration. The reason for that is that we have borrowed biomechanics from general orthopedics, and those biomechanics are not sufficient to explain which one of these procedures is superior to the other procedures. It is not that simple.

There might be a procedure that is superior to the other procedures; however, it is not feasible to perform that procedure due to anatomical structures. That is why I say that it should be left to the surgeon who performs the surgery to make that decision, and left for the patient to feel comfortable with the surgeon performing the surgery. I always tell my patients that I welcome second opinions.

Risks and Benefits

I divide the risks of fusion surgeries into two categories. One category is the risks that are inherent to the anatomy. These include nerve damage, vessel damage, or dural tear. Dura is the sac that the nerves and neural structures are covered and protected by. The brain is floating in the skull in spinal fluid, covered by arachnoid membrane and the dural sac. If this sac, which is paper thin, gets nicked, it can leak fluid, and the treatment for that is oversewing the sac and stopping the leakage.

When we do spine surgery, we are millimeters away from the nerves. There can be damage if the nerve is compressed directly or indirectly during the surgery.

Another risk would be damage to the large vessels in front of the vertebrae in the lumbar spine. The aorta, iliac vessels, and arteries are usually robust structures, and their walls are thick and strong. They normally do not get damaged. However, the large veins, including the vena cava, are very thin-walled structures. There is plenty of blood in the inferior vena cava. That is one of the reasons that I use an approach surgeon for my surgeries. If there is an adverse event during the surgery, I would rather have someone used to dealing with those problems next to me.

In terms of the cervical spine, one of the risks is damage to the voice box. If the surgeon is overzealous or the surgery is long, nerve damage can affect the voice. The other problem related to cervical anatomy is esophageal damage. This is something that we think comes from extended compression of the esophagus. We do not know exactly how it happens, so we have a difficult time avoiding it. With this injury, the patient develops swallowing difficulty after surgery. Swallowing difficulty that bothers the patient is rare, and it is more like a nuisance to the patient. Sometimes a patient reports that they must physically think to push down a piece of steak. Major swallowing difficulty is very rare. These are the risks that are based on the anatomy where we are performing the surgery.

The second group of risks are inherent to the surgery itself. When we are doing the surgery, the patient is asleep and cannot tell us if the nerves have been decompressed enough or need further decompression. The time in the operating room needs to be minimized for multiple reasons. With the patient asleep for an extended period, there are high risks for unwanted events, such as blood clots in the leg, which can be very dangerous, or pneumonia. Surgery should be performed to get the patient off the table in a reasonable time.

One of the main risks of surgery is that the surgery might not work. When I see a problem on the MRI that explains the patient's symptoms, my job is to fix that problem. However, I do not have control over what happens after that. I have done thousands of surgeries in my practice. You hope the pain they were suffering from before the surgery has resolved. But since the patient is asleep during the procedure, they cannot tell me if I have done the right surgery.

The second risk inherent to fusion surgery is nonunion. With fusion surgery, you are trying to make a bridge to turn the two bones into one bone. Even with the best carpentry and best work, that might not happen. In large part, it depends on the patient's biology, which the surgeon does not have control over. Sometimes this fusion might not solidify.

The entire goal of this book is to bring to light that, so far, we as surgeons have not used proper devices and techniques to increase fusion rates. The goal is to increase the fusion rate so that more people can have their bones heal together and achieve pain relief.

The bones' chances of not healing are 10% to 25%, depending on what technique is used and which research you read. Therefore, it is not minimal. If nonunion happens, we are obligated to go back and redo the surgery to get that area to heal.

Not all nonunions are painful, though most are. I have had patients who have done fusion surgery, and I could not see a solid fusion mass on the postoperative CT scan; however, the patient was thrilled with the surgery. That happens quite a bit. In these cases, even though I cannot see evidence of a fusion, there is no need to go back and perform another surgery to get the area to fuse because the patient is not having any symptoms. After all, our goal is to treat the patient's pain and not the imaging studies.

To become a surgical candidate, the patient must usually have pain that doesn't get better with therapy and injections. In this situation, the patient has tried everything available in terms of nonoperative care, and they have not had significant pain relief. If the pain is intolerable, the patient can exercise their right to go to the next option: surgical intervention.

The next necessary step is for the surgeon to identify a problem that he believes explains the patient's symptoms. I divide my patients into two categories: simple and complex. A simple patient will have one or two bad discs. A complex patient will have three or more discs that are bad. This is because when a patient goes from two bad discs to three, the problem goes from a localized to a regional problem.

If a patient's problem is a localized area, they do very well with a one- or two-level fusion. There is a 40 percent chance of a pain-free or a relatively pain-free back—almost like a brand-new back—and a 45 percent chance for a significant decrease in the pain, but they would always have residual pain that simply would not go away. They would have a 10% to 15% chance that the surgery would not work for them.

If the injured discs span a larger area and involve three or four discs, the patient will require a large, extended fusion. In these cases, it is essential to discuss with the patient what can be expected after surgery.

Often, if a patient is dissatisfied with surgery, it's because the surgeon did not take enough time to explain exactly what could happen after the procedure. The patient needs to have a realistic expectation of the surgery when the problem is regional. In these situations, I tell my patients that the goal of the surgery is really to stabilize the back so it does not worsen. In these cases, even though it might appear to the patient that they are not significantly better, the true benefit of the surgery— which is stopping the pain, numbness and tingling, or weakness from getting worse—cannot be seen. That is an essential point for the patient to understand.

Shotgun Surgery – Very Important – Must Read

Statistically speaking, it is very hard for me to believe that all the discs can hurt the patient equally. More likely than not, it is one disc that is hurting the patient more than any others. That is because the discs are independent structures not connected to each other. Now, I am not saying that only one disc can hurt at a time. I am saying that the bad pain that pushes the patient toward surgery is most likely coming from one source, and that is very difficult to identify when we see three or four discs that can potentially be the source. In these situations, of course, the surgeon wants to fix the patient and treat their pain. Therefore, we tend to fix all of the discs that could potentially contribute to the patient's pain. I call this "shotgun surgery."

Why do I want to make a big deal out of this topic? Because the bigger the surgery we perform, the bigger the consequences for the patient's future. There is a significant difference between a one-level fusion and a three-level fusion in terms of morbidity that the surgery causes the patient. With the concept of shotgun surgery, in which the surgeon tries to address all the issues that could be contributing to the patient's pain, the patient is actually getting a surgery that they do not need.

Unfortunately, at this time we do not have a test or study that can tell us where the pain is coming from. There is a way that we can estimate its origin based on the patient's complaints and the pain behavior. Every little thing the patient tells me is a clue. The way the patient sits on a chair is a clue. The way the patient gets up from a chair is a clue. The way the patient walks is a clue. The distribution of the pain pattern is also a clue. The surgeon has to consider all these complaints to determine the possible location of the pain generation with a little more confidence. This ability comes to the surgeon through decades of practice; some surgeons never achieve this level of intuition because they rely heavily on physician assistants to run their practices.

This topic is important in a younger, more active population in the productive stage of life. Once a patient enters retirement age, preserving function is not as critical. However, with someone young—in their thirties or forties, at the peak of their career—the goal of the spine surgeon should be to avoid very large surgery so that the patient does not get derailed from their career path. I will give you an example.

In 2018, I had a patient who was a thirty-three-year-old mother of two who had been involved in a motor vehicle accident and was suffering from severe neck and arm pain. The patient had a badly injured disc at the level of C5-6 and a minor tear at the level of C4-5. The patient was very eager to return to work because she had a family to support, and a mortgage and car payment.

I understand this situation. I support my family as well. However, as a responsible spine surgeon, I always look at the bigger picture. The picture I look at is what I can do today so my patient will be in the best shape possible at the age of seventy. I will consider how easy or hard life will be for them.

This patient had tried nonoperative care, which had not helped her. So, she was contemplating surgery. I told her that I believed in my heart that the best option for her would be a disc arthroplasty at the level of C5-6 because she was so young. I knew that her pain was originating from the disc at the level of C5-6 based on my examination and the patient's complaint.

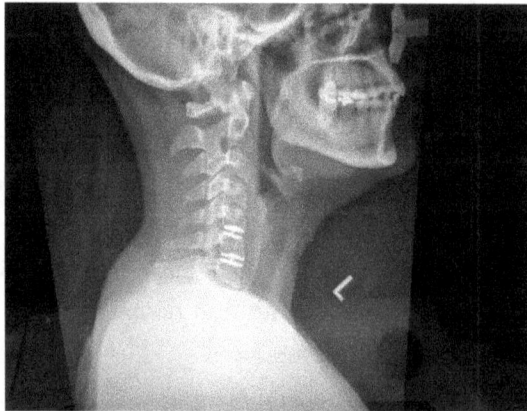

Figure 24: Cervical Disc Replacement - Arthroplasty

She needed to understand there was a chance that there could be some pain coming from the C4-5 disc space, and she might require a second surgery to address this if her pain did not resolve with one-level disc arthroplasty at the level of C5-6. I told her that a one-level disc arthroplasty would not throw the biomechanics of the spine off balance. I offered her surgery with the potential 80 percent chance of success and little downside. I told her that a two-level disc replacement would give her an 80% to 90% chance of success, but a two-level disc replacement would affect the biomechanics of her spine forever. Going from a one-level disc replacement to a two-level disc replacement changes the biomechanics of the spine—not in a good way. (I will explain disc replacement versus fusion surgery in the next section.)

The patient did not like that idea. She wanted one surgery and to go on with her life. She got a second opinion from another surgeon who was in practice for only a few years. The other surgeon advised a two-level anterior cervical discectomy and fusion as the most appropriate surgery. That is precisely what I call shotgun surgery. I told the patient that I did not disagree with that surgeon. I could do a two-level surgery, and we could argue about fusion versus disc replacement forever.

A two-level surgery, either fusion or disc replacement, would help the patient significantly; however, the patient would be entering unchartered territory. I told her that the disc at the level of C5-6 is the most commonly injured and painful disc; it was at fault in probably 80 percent of my patients who suffered from a neck injury. I was confident, based on my detailed evaluation of the patient and the look of her MRI, that it was the C5-6 disc that was bothering her. But the two-level surgery in a thirty-three-year-old would have significant implications down the road, leading to even more surgeries.

There is a threshold in the biomechanics of the cervical spine and the lumbar spine. If this threshold is not crossed during the surgery, the patient's future will not be affected. If that threshold is crossed in terms of the magnitude of the surgery, the future course for the patient will be affected and most likely accelerate the demise of the spine's function. We do not know exactly where this threshold is. That is what experience brings to a spine surgeon.

The surgeon that gave the second opinion was only a few years into his practice. That is where I was, too, at that point in my career. It took me twenty years to make decisions that would not alter patient's course toward the worst outcome. This is a very important concept that I want my readers to understand. I totally understand that no patient wants to hear or even imagine a possible second surgery. Everyone wants to go back to work and be able to support their family as soon as possible, but spine surgery is much more complex. With the diagnostic studies currently available to us, that expectation is sometimes unachievable. We are just starting to understand the complex biomechanics of the spine. We are just starting to understand what the surgery itself is doing to the patient. As I have mentioned, spine surgery is a very young field. What makes this even more difficult is the different presentation of every patient and the different circumstances each patient is in.

I explained to this patient that it is a very easy decision to do a two-level surgery in all the areas that could possibly generate the pain. If the patient does not get better for some reason, the surgeon has done all he could to help the patient. Nobody would blame the surgeon for decisions made. However, it is an extremely gutsy decision by me to suggest a smaller, one-level surgery, understanding that there is the possibility of the need for a second surgery. In this case, if the patient does not get better from surgery, the surgeon would be under a tremendous amount of scrutiny for not performing adequate surgery.

Now, I would like to be completely honest with my readers. Some people might accuse me of driving the patient toward a path of doing more surgeries. I assure you that is not the case. There is nothing in this world worse for a spine surgeon than a patient that is not better after surgery. When I do surgery and the patient is not better afterward, I do not send them to pain management to never see them again. The patient gets into my mind, and I constantly think about them. The patient becomes a source of stress for me. If the patient is not better after a second surgery, we are in a very difficult situation. There is a tremendous amount of pressure on the surgeon to make sure the second surgery will help the patient.

The thirty-three-year-old patient did not like the idea that I presented to her. She went to the younger surgeon for a two-level surgery. I felt that was a travesty. I do not remember doing a two-level surgery on anyone younger than forty years of age in my practice. However, I do not condemn the other surgeon because I would have probably done the same surgery if this patient presented to my practice when I was at that stage of my career.

The thirty-three-year-old ended up with a two-level fusion, and she has no idea what is waiting for her in the future. There is a very strong chance she will need her entire cervical spine fused by the age of sixty. I remember telling this patient that even if she did not get better with the first surgery and required a second surgery, I would not regret my decision based on my assessment of the patient.

I remember when I had just started my practice in 2002, I would see the surgeries that the more established surgeons were doing, and they were much smaller surgeries. I started doing long, complex fusions. I remember telling myself that these established surgeons were probably not well trained in terms of spine surgery, as it was a very new subspecialty. Two decades into my practice, I find myself in the same situation as the established surgeons at that time, trying to go out of my way to perform smaller surgeries. Throughout the last two decades of my career, with close monitoring of my patients, I can see what a large surgery can do to them in terms of limiting their activities.

Spine surgery is a subspecialty of other surgeries. As I have mentioned multiple times, it is a very young field. In orthopedic surgery, our exposure to spine surgery is very minimal. Even in the fellowship that I received, the important thing that I learned was how to perform the surgeries and become a safe, efficient surgeon. After two decades of practice, I realize that the most important aspect of spine surgery is a full assessment of the patient to diagnose where the pain is coming from. We get very minimal exposure to this aspect of spine surgery because, as residents, we spend most of our time in the operating room. That is what most residents would like to do, since managing a clinic and seeing patients is the most boring part of the residency.

During the first decade of my practice, I was very busy performing complex surgeries, and for a time, I was operating four days a week. I used the shotgun approach for my surgeries. It was not until I entered the second decade of my practice that I started asking questions and looking at what we did and our principles with a much more critical eye. Now I realize that the training of a spine surgeon should be to try to do the smallest surgery with the most preservation of tissue and function.

For the first part of my practice, I was a technician more than a spine surgeon. I would base my entire decision-making process on the visual aspect of the MRI. Now what I see on the MRI is only part of the puzzle. Every little thing the patient tells me is very valuable to me. Every complaint, and even the patient's appearance, can contribute valuable information. Some surgeons remain technicians throughout their entire careers, and they do not transition toward the next stage. With the current heavy industry influence on spine surgery, performing smaller surgeries is not even in the prospects of spine surgery teachings.

To perform smaller surgeries by identifying the pain generators, we need better diagnostic tests. We have discography, a diagnostic test in which the patient is completely awake. The examiner places long needles through the skin into the discs under X-rays. The examiner injects the discs sequentially. The patient is not aware of which disc is being injected. If the healthy disc is injected, the examiner asks the patient if there is any pain. If the patient states there is no pain at this location but expresses pain with the injection of the diseased disc, that is a positive finding. The second question from the examiner is if this is the pain that they normally experience. If the answer is yes, then that is a positive finding.

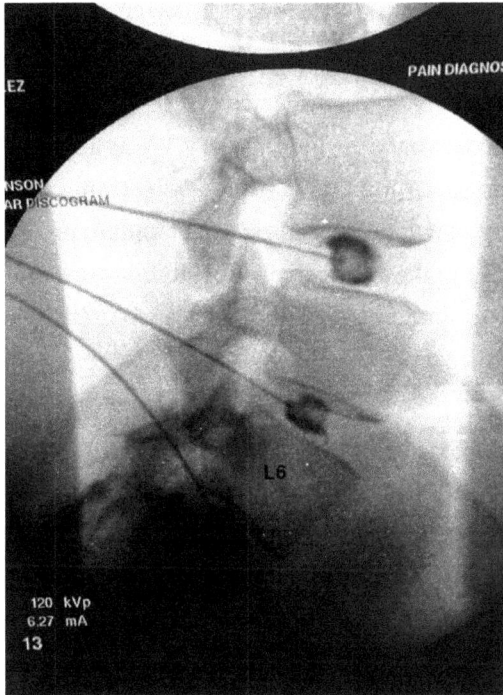

Figure 25: Discography Example

This test is very controversial due to the fact that a good test depends on how skilled the examiner is. At this time, this is the only test available to us, and there is absolutely no other test that can show us where the pain is coming from.

We cannot wait around for an invention that may or may not come. We have to progress as spine surgeons and improve our surgeries. This starts with proper training of residents. Then, as a specialty, we have to have the right attitude toward what is best for the patient, which is to preserve as much function as possible.

Also, a very important aspect of this movement is patient education. The public needs to have a better understanding of what we do in spine surgery. At this time, the only expectation of the public is to have one surgery that will eliminate the pain completely. Patients need to understand that this expectation can push the surgeon toward doing a very large surgery. It all starts with patient education and decreasing the influence of the industry in spine surgery.

We are at a crossroads in spine surgery. We as a specialty will need to decide whether we are going to continue performing shotgun surgeries, in which case there will be no improvement and no progress in our field, or we are going to make a collective effort to fine-tune spine surgery and perform only the surgery that the patient absolutely needs. That is the future of spine surgery.

Disc Arthroplasty

When spine surgeons started doing fusion surgeries, we also started seeing patients coming back a few years later with the disc adjacent to the level that was fused going bad. We started looking at this phenomenon a little bit closer. The argument was that the first disc went bad, and once it was fused, it placed pressure on the disc next to it, which had now gone bad because of the fusion.

The cervical spine and the lumbar spine each have a specific range of motion. Once one level is fused, the stress of motion is spread between a fewer number of discs. This means there is more stress distributed to each disc that is not fused. We believe there is a phenomenon called *adjacent-level disease* that can accelerate degeneration and damage the disc next to a fused disc. There is intense research being done to answer that question.

This was the phenomenon that made spine surgeons start thinking about possible alternatives. One alternative was not to fuse the disc and see if we could replace it with a prosthesis that could move and duplicate the disc's motion. We currently have discs available for the cervical spine and the lumbar spine. We have had a decent amount of information from these surgeries. However, there is a significant difference between cervical and lumbar disc replacement surgeries.

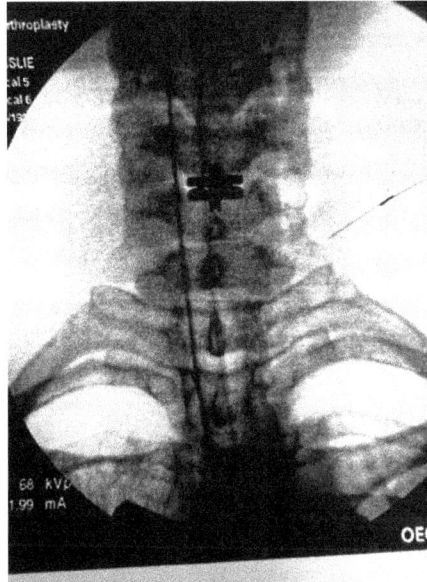

Figure 26: Disc Replacement Prosthesis

The first disc replacement that became available was for the lumbar spine. I am not sure about the regulations in Europe, but it was about ten years ahead of the United States in terms of disc replacement. They did have fair results, so we started doing this in America, too. We quickly found the results of the disc replacement in the lumbar spine were not good. We blamed the specific type of disc that became available in the United States first. We gave disc replacement a second go with a better prosthesis. However, that did not turn out so great, either.

At this time, lumbar disc replacements come in and out of the field. I feel it is the drug companies that are forcing disc replacements in the lumbar spine back into the field.

In the lumbar spine, stability is much more important than the range of motion, meaning fusion is better than disc replacement in the lower back. A disc replacement prosthesis is a device that is designed to duplicate the motion of the disc. The disc is a very complex structure and has two functions: to promote motion, and to restrict excessive motion by stabilizing the two vertebrae against each other. The disc is a very strong structure that connects to the vertebra above and the vertebra below. With a disc replacement, there is a free motion between the two vertebrae and absolutely no connection between the two halves of the prosthesis. This causes significant problems. Once we replace the disc, this excessive motion causes significant stretch and stress on the facet joints.

We really do not understand the long-term consequences of disc replacement. But one thing is for sure: nothing in the body that moves lasts the lifetime of the patient. At some point, these prostheses break down, and we must do revision surgery, which would then be a fusion.

I do not want to bore the readers with the details of a disc replacement. After about fifteen years of these discs being available in the United States, I do not believe in the effectiveness of disc replacement in the lumbar spine, and I have never performed this procedure. It is not a very difficult surgery.

There were significant failures in the disc replacement in the lumbar spine. I believe that has something to do with the amount of force that the lumbar spine must endure. In the cervical spine, we are talking about only the weight of the head, but in the lumbar spine, we are talking about the entire weight of the torso, upper extremities, and the head. In the cervical spine, there's a much smaller lever arm, while in the lumbar spine, the lever arm is very long. Therefore, in the lumbar spine, there is significant stress on the replacement disc where metal and bone contact each other, causing substantial failures.

The other important problem with disc replacement in the lumbar spine is anatomy. To perform a disc replacement in the lumbar spine, we must get the vena cava, the biggest vein in the body, out of the way.

This vena cava is paper thin and scars down once you perform surgery. If there is a failure of a disc, it is extremely hard to go back and try to revise that disc replacement due to that scarring. It is very difficult to move the vena cava out of the way and almost impossible sometimes. If you tear the vena cava, there is a risk of death, which has occurred.

Based on what we know now, I consider performing lumbar disc replacement a poor decision on the part of surgeons. Those that continue performing lumbar disc replacement do not truly understand the specific biomechanics of the spine. If we have to choose between stability or motion for a spine in a diseased state, there is no question that stability is far more important than motion in the lumbar spine.

The cervical spine is very different. In the cervical spine, my surgeries are divided equally. About half of the time, I perform a fusion surgery, and about half of the time, I perform disc replacement surgery. The results in the cervical spine are good, and patients are happy. If I have a patient older than fifty-five, I tend to perform a fusion surgery. Once the fusion solidifies, it will last the patient's entire life. I perform disc replacement surgery for a patient younger than forty-five to avoid junctional disc damage. Between the ages of forty-five and fifty-five, it is a toss-up. I explain the disc replacement and fusion surgery options in detail and get the patient involved in the decision. Some patients do not want their bones fused, and in that case, we perform disc replacement surgery. However, some patients would like to have surgery with the best possible outcome and, in that case, we proceed with fusion surgery.

The great majority of research on disc replacements are paid for by device manufacturing companies. The results of these studies are impressive. The disc replacement devices are able to do everything that they have advertised. They control pain better than fusion and they stop adjacent levels from going bad.

By giving patients forms to complete in terms of their satisfaction after fusion surgery or disc replacement surgery in the cervical spine, I do not doubt that both groups will give high marks to their surgery.

However, I believe that if the two patients—disc replacement and fusion—are placed in one room to talk to each other, most disc replacement patients would rather have had fusion surgery. That is because disc replacement gets rid of most of the severe pain; however, some minor pain in the form of a nuisance, like a twinge here and there or occasional minor headaches, do linger. The number of patients who achieve complete pain relief is more common in fusion surgery than in disc replacement surgery. In a young person, I would perform disc replacement over fusion surgery to preserve their cervical range of motion, which remains an intense research area.

CHAPTER FIVE

~

The Evidence Against
Pedicle Screws

One of the most common surgeries we do is spinal fusion. We use a device called a *pedicle screw* in pretty much every fusion that we do. In this chapter, I will be presenting evidence, based on papers that have been published in leading journals of spine surgery, that pedicle screws do not work. This is clear evidence that has been completely ignored.

Just one article, published by one surgeon, based on a study that was apparently abandoned in the middle and never finished, shows that the pedicle screws work beautifully. This one article has unfortunately become the gold standard and basis of what we do today in the world of spine surgery.

The studies I will present were conducted with the purpose of evaluating the current practice of spine surgery. The core question that they were trying to answer was whether the equipment that we use in spine surgery currently is helping our patients or is completely worthless. At the center of this question is the pedicle screw.

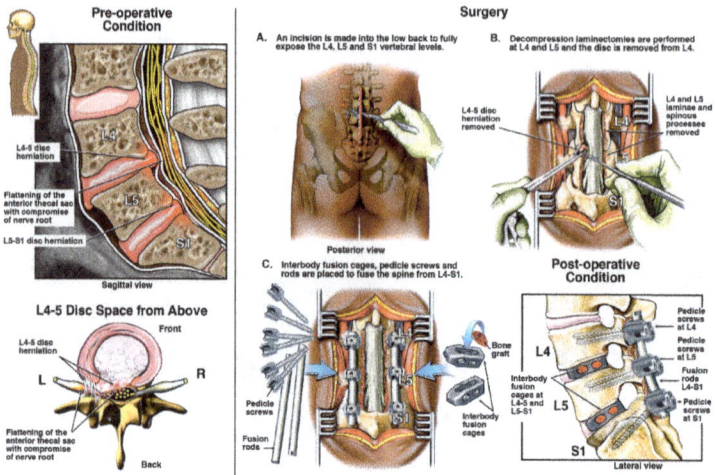

Figure 27: L4-5 and L5-S1 Disc Herniations with Posterior Discectomy Fusion

I've mentioned this device several times in this book, but I will detail its use again here. A pedicle screw is a very large screw that is inserted from the back of the spine toward the front of the spine. It is inserted through the middle of a bone column called a *pedicle*. Then these screws are connected to each other by rods. Each vertebra has two pedicles on each side. These pedicles form a column of bone that connects the vertebral body to the posterior structures called the *lamina*. If you can imagine, the pedicle is a big tube with the outside bone being cortical and the inside bone being spongy cancellous bone.

The entire reason I am writing this book is for my audience and patients with back pain to understand the fact that after millions of screws have been implanted over the past three and a half decades, spine surgeons have not been able to show that the addition of these screws translates into benefit in the outcome of our spine surgeries. But the problem is not just one device. This problem is just the tip of the iceberg. The real problem is our understanding and core philosophy of spine surgery. The problem is much deeper.

When pedicle screws first appeared in spine surgery in the mid-1980s and early 1990s, there was significant skepticism surrounding their use. The initial results were not good, and there were lawsuits secondary to bad outcomes—some 7,000 of them, according to the *Washington Post*. The FDA actually initially refused to approve the use of the screws for spinal surgery.

In 1993, an article was published in the journal *Spine* by a surgeon named Dr. Thomas Zdeblick. He was the only author of the article, which essentially claimed that pedicle screws improved fusion rates and outcomes beautifully. This was a turning point in the entire world of spine surgery. As I write this chapter, searching online for "Zdeblick spine fusion" shows that this article has been referenced by 1,080 other articles. It is the most referenced article in the entire world of spine surgery. In my opinion, there are significant problems with this article, which I will dissect one by one later in this chapter.

In the late 1990s and early 2000s, six independent articles (see page 110) appeared in three prominent medical journals regarding the use of pedicle screws. These studies are multicenter, multinational, and published in reputable journals. Some of these articles won awards for their quality of research and how they were conducted. They all reached the same conclusion: pedicle screws did not increase fusion rate and did not have any impact on the outcome of surgery. They clearly showed that surgeries without the use of expensive hardware had as good an outcome as the very expensive surgeries using the screws as an adjunct. In stark opposition to the article published by Dr. Zdeblick, these articles showed that pedicle screws are completely useless. These articles are very well known to spine surgeons and leaders of the field.

However, right around the same time these articles were being published, the use of pedicle screws skyrocketed, and their use became the gold standard in performing fusions of the spine. This is a big deal. Placing screws is not a benign event.

There are multiple layers of problems with the insertion of pedicle screws in the spine. One issue, which is the most obvious, is the cost. Screws are very expensive, sometimes in excess of $1,000 each. In addition, significant supporting elements are required for implantation. A radiology technician is necessary to run the live imaging used to guide the placement of the screws. A neurophysiologist or electrophysiologist is also necessary in the operating room. This specialist monitors the nerves of the patient throughout the surgery so the surgeon does not insert the screw close to the nerves. After the surgery, X-rays and CT scans are required to confirm the position of the screws. The addition of screws leads to increased time of surgery, increased blood loss, and the possibility of nerve damage, which translates to higher complication rates. Some of these complications can be very serious and even lethal. And it does not end there.

To insert the screws, the surgeon must make an extensive dissection of paraspinal muscles off the spine. The surgeon basically dissects the muscle off the bone from corner to corner. Research has shown that this amount of dissection kills a significant amount of the paraspinal muscles and creates scar tissue. This leads to significant dysfunction of these muscles, which are very important for recovery and the outcome of the surgery. It is almost as though the surgery replaces one pain with a different type of pain. We do this surgery when the patient is experiencing sharp, stabbing pain that is intolerable and not controlled with pain medication, which is then replaced by a pain that is dull and achy but manageable with pain medication. We didn't eliminate pain; we simply replaced one kind with another, but patients were very happy.

With six multicenter, multinational research articles indicating that these screws do not work in terms of increasing fusion rate or improving outcome, and with only one article written by one individual that was apparently abandoned in the middle and never finished, the big question is why the use of pedicle screws skyrocketed and became the standard of care when performing spinal fusion. I have asked this question of many leaders in the field of spine surgery, and I get the same answer from everyone: It is just a statistical glitch that we have not been able to show with research that these pedicle screws do work. I am writing this book in order to explain that there is a very serious and deep reason that research has shown that these screws do not work.

It is absolutely baffling to me that leaders in the field blame a statistical glitch for a finding by research papers whose answers they are not happy with. We are scientists, surgeons, and doctors. We cannot be satisfied with a statistical glitch as an explanation, or at least I am not satisfied with it. As a matter of fact, in the next three chapters, I will be explaining why I believe all the follow-up research is correct and how the heavy influence of industry has turned spine surgery into what—in my mind, and in my interpretation of the published research—is the biggest scam in the history of medicine.

As a subspecialty of orthopedic surgery, we have used biomechanics appropriate for orthopedics to treat spine surgery patients. The truth is that spine surgery was never meant to be a subspecialty of orthopedic surgery or neurosurgery. Spine surgery is a much more complex field than general orthopedics. Spine surgery has its own rules and biomechanics that need to be studied, developed, and applied to the treatment of spine conditions. That is exactly what I have been working on nonstop for the past six years. I will explain that in Chapter Eight.

Selection of Papers

I would like to explain how I selected these papers. When you are trying to answer a certain question and run a study, you can conduct the study in different ways.

For example, a retrospective study is when a large number of cases have been completed, and you look back at the patients who have received a certain type of treatment and review their charts to see how they did. A retrospective study is pretty much a chart review study.

These studies are notorious for being very susceptible to bias, because the results depend on who is selected to enter the study. With this type of study, you are able to pretty much publish whatever you want, as long as you select the patients with your desired outcome. There are a lot of retrospective studies in the world of spine surgery, and I consider these to have very low power in terms of their value.

The gold standard type of study for investigating the effectiveness of a certain type of treatment is a prospective, randomized study. *Prospective* means that you start from one point in time and analyze data going forward. *Randomized* means that there is a group that receives the treatment and a control group that does not receive the treatment that you are evaluating. The patients are assigned to each group on a random basis. The experiment has a predetermined length of time, from a few months to a few years.The results are subjected to a rigorous statistical analysis to determine any difference between the two groups.

When I reviewed the literature, I considered the recommendations by the Congress of Neurological Surgeons, the North American Spine Society, and the general literature, and I picked only prospective, randomized studies that were very well known to the spine community so there would be no question as to the validity of these studies.

The Zdeblick Study

First, I will discuss in detail the only prospective, randomized study to this date that showed that pedicle screws work beautifully. This is the 1993 paper by Dr. Zdeblick published in the journal *Spine*.

This study was advertised as a prospective, randomized study of lumbar fusion. Dr. Zdeblick had three groups in this study, each with about forty patients. One group did not receive any instrumentation along with their fusion of the lumbar spine. The second group received instrumentation that was not very rigid. The third group received a very rigid pedicle screw and rod system as an adjunct to their fusion. Dr. Zdeblick claimed that the fusion rate went up as the rigidity of the construct went up. There was also clear evidence that as a more rigid instrumentation system was used, the outcome of the surgeries improved significantly.

Everything that we do in the world of spine surgery as of today tracks back to this one paper. Without this paper, we would have absolutely nothing to show that the pedicle screw and rod system accomplishes anything whatsoever. That is how important this paper is.

There are, in my opinion, significant problems with this paper, all of which Dr. Zdeblick has denied. The first and most disturbing issue is, again in my opinion, that this paper was published as a preliminary report on June 15, 1993. I spent about a year and a half looking for the final results in the literature, and I was baffled that l could not find a final report or a follow-up report. When I was at a conference, I spoke to a professor from a major Midwest medical school about this, and he told me that this preliminary report is the only thing available, and there is no final report. Apparently, this experiment was abandoned in the middle, and Dr. Zdeblick never finished it. If you read the paper online from the National Library of Medicine, you will see that it still says "Preliminary results" even though it was published nearly thirty years ago.

I went through rigorous training in my orthopedic surgery and spine fellowship, and I have gone to conferences at least twice a year through-out my career. I have seen how award-winning papers are often dissected and criticized. However, to this day, I have never heard that a preliminary report would satisfy the scientific criteria for completeness and validity. I believe this is true for any specialty or field.

As an instrument-rated aircraft pilot, I read many preliminary reports, and the final verdict is often different than the preliminary report. When I order a medical test and get a preliminary read back, I do not accept it as the final say; I always wait for the official report. I do not understand how an unfinished experiment has become the quintessential anchor for an entire field, in this case, the field of spine surgery. I am baffled that this study has been referenced in more than

1,080 articles. It is hard for me to imagine these authors never raised the question of where the final report is. If the scientific standard is so low that we accept a preliminary report as the final say, why would we bother to ever write the final report? Why do we call a report "preliminary" to begin with? For me, a preliminary report means that the results are subject to change, and simply more work needs to be done and more data needs to be turned in.

What I believe is the second very disturbing problem with this study is actually mentioned inside the abstract of the study. This study included 124 patients. There were three groups, and each group consisted of roughly forty patients. It was a randomized study, and that means the patients were assigned to each group on a random basis. However, Dr. Zdeblick states that nine patients who were originally assigned to groups two or three (which were supposed to receive instruments or hardware) were moved to group one (the group that was not supposed to receive the hardware) intraoperatively. He mentions that this change was due to the identification of severe osteopenia (weak bone) and the determination that the pedicle screw purchase was poor. (Dr. Zdeblick denied any wrongdoing in this re-assignment.)

That is a big deal. The whole idea of a study being randomized is so that the patients are randomly assigned to a group, and they are supposed to stay in that group. They are supposed to receive the treatment in question, and they must stay in that group to eventually find out if that treatment worked for them. Dr. Zdeblick transferred nine patients to a group that was not supposed to receive the hardware. It is my opinion that this is not just sloppy research; it could be viewed as tampering. Once he found out that these patients were not going to do well because the pedicle screws failed intraoperatively, he transferred those patients to a group that was not supposed to receive hardware. This does not seem right. A scientist cannot find out something negative about a patient then transfer them to another group. That could be seen as the ultimate way of showing bias.

I can see a situation that calls for doing what is appropriate for the patient intraoperatively, regardless of the study. However, at that point, the proper methodology would be to exclude that patient from the experiment. This is not ideal, but it is not horrible. By transferring those patients to another group, knowing that their bone quality was poor, I believe it is taking sides in terms of which group Dr. Zdeblick wanted to do well and which group he did not want to do well. In a group of forty patients, nine patients can make a big difference in the outcome, as it is nearly 25 percent of the total group. (Dr. Zdeblick has denied any wrongdoing in the transferring of these patients in the study.)

Therefore, in my opinion, this study is not a randomized study. In actuality, to this day, I do not believe that we have a prospective, randomized study showing that the pedicle screws work; Dr. Zdeblick's paper calls itself "randomized" but, in my opinion, it seems at odds with how a truly randomized trial would be conducted. (Again, Dr. Zdeblick has denied any issues with his research methodology.)

The third problem with this study is regarding Dr. Zdeblick's conduct. According to a US Senate probe, Dr. Zdeblick was involved in at least two important studies published in 2002 and 2003. At the time, he was conducting experiments with a product he helped to develop with a company called Medtronic. According to a US Department of Justice investigation and two US Senate committee probes, Medtronic paid him $34.168 million between 1996 and 2010. (The details are found in the "Staff Report on Medtronic's Influence on Infuse Clinical Studies," prepared by the Staff of the Committee on Finance—United States Senate, October 2012.)

The US Senate probe stated the following: "Medtronic Employees Were Substantively Involved in Producing Journal Articles Authored by the Company's Physician Consultants. A review of the documents Medtronic provided to the Committee demonstrates that Medtronic employees, including employees working for its marketing department, collaborated with physician authors, many of whom had significant financial relationships with Medtronic, to draft the following studies:".

The report then cited the seven studies, including two coauthored by Dr. Zdeblick. (Note that Dr. Zdeblick denied any wrongdoing. In a news release, Medtronic said, "Medtronic vigorously disagrees with any suggestion that the company improperly influenced or authored any of the peer-reviewed published manuscripts discussed in the report, or that Medtronic intended to under-report adverse events.")

If you search "Dr. Carragee of Spine journal" in YouTube, you will find a video from 2012. CNN sent a reporter to the NASS Annual Meeting to find and interview Dr. Zdeblick, but he was not there, even though he was scheduled to appear. CNN said in its broadcast that they wanted to ask him why Medtronic paid him $34 million. When he failed to show, CNN reported that they called him, but Dr. Zdeblick did not return their calls. Instead, CNN interviewed Dr. Carragee, a professor at Stanford University and the editor of *Spine*, who said, "We didn't live up to the expectations of the profession."

Once a researcher's ethics come into question because of a study, I believe this could put the researcher's previous studies under question and could discredit them.

I believe there is a fourth big problem with Dr. Zdeblick's study: the circumstances in 1993, when his paper was published. The following excerpt is from court filings in the US District Court for the Eastern District of Pennsylvania In Re: Orthopedic Bone Screw Products Liability Litigation. AcroMed was a medical device company that was acquired in 1998 by DePuy and subsequently by Johnson & Johnson. Sofamor Danek was a non-settling defendant in the case. In 1999, Sofamor Danek Group merged with Medtronic and eventually became Medtronic's Spinal and Biologics business unit.

> Sofamor Danek and AcroMed have similar bone screw products that are the subject of this litigation and the "litigation experience of Sofamor Danek has been somewhat similar to the recent litigation experience of AcroMed."

AcroMed is a manufacturer of orthopedic bone screws that in recent years have been used by surgeons in spinal fusion surgery. (Rountree Decl. ¶¶ 3-5). In December 1993, the ABC News program *20/20* featured a story on the screws and their use in the pedicle of the spine. (Werder Decl. ¶ 4). After that broadcast, thousands of people who had undergone spinal fusion surgery involving pedicle screws filed suit against AcroMed and other pedicle screw manufacturers. In August 1994, the Judicial Panel on Multidistrict Litigation transferred all cases pending in federal trial courts against manufacturers of pedicle screws to this court for pretrial purposes pursuant to 28 U.S.C. § 1407.

The lawsuit was settled without any admissions.

According to the *Los Angeles Times*, the class-action lawsuit was brought by 3,000 people who said they had suffered from the use of pedicle screws. The suit was ultimately settled for $100 million. AcroMed said in a statement, "We have taken this action despite our firm belief that claims arising from the use of these devices in spinal fusion surgeries are without merit."

The FDA was refusing to approve the use of these pedicle screws for spinal operations at that time. The screws were eventually approved in 1985 only for general bone surgery, not lower back surgery. But once that approval was granted, surgeons used the product "off-label," essentially as a backdoor strategy.

According to a March 29, 1996, article published in the *Washington Post*, entitled "The Tangled Path of FDA Review":

> The industry developed financial ties with about 200 spine surgeons and these doctors provided services that ranged from consulting work to spreading the word about the pedicle device's utility, the lawyers allege. According to their FDA comment, surgeons made more than 1,000 appearances at some 230 professional meetings

where pedicle screw devices were demonstrated. All told, the law-yers allege, the industry paid out more than $29 million in cash and gave out stock or stock options. The firms also donated $5 million to medical institutions where these doctors work, their FDA com-ment asserts.

It's a fascinating case study in how big medical-device companies seemingly wielded influence to push their agenda despite lawsuits, much-criticized clinical trials, and likely conflicts of interest. In 1994, an FDA advisory panel voted to recommend that the pedicle screw be reclassified as a less risky device that did not require premarket stud-ies. Effective December 30, 2016, the FDA officially reclassified pedicle screw systems as a Class II/special controls device instead of as a high-er-risk Class III device.

The information about the use of pedicle screws in spinal surgery was widely reported by major reputable sources, including the *Washing-ton Post*, the *Los Angeles Times*, CNN, and ABC News, as noted above, and yet there were (and still are) so many unanswered questions. Why was this paper published as a preliminary report, and what was the rush? What was happening at the time that Dr. Zdeblick decided to publish this paper as a preliminary report? Did the publication of this study coincide with the lawsuits in the late 1990s? Dr. Zdeblick reportedly received $34 million from Medtronic between 1996 and 2010, purport-edly as royalties for other devices he invented and for consulting fees. Did the payments coincide with the lawsuits disappearing? The other important fact is that Dr. Zdeblick's work has not yet been duplicated, even after multiple studies.

According to a 2006 article published in The [ital.] *New York Times*, a whistleblower suit was filed against Medtronic in US District Court by a former Medtronic employee. It accused the company of paying spine surgeons "excessive remuneration, unlawful perquisites, and bribes in other forms for purchasing goods and medical devices." The suit was dismissed in 2009 by a federal judge in Massachusetts, and there were no findings against Medtronic.

The *New York Times* article from 2006 alleged that Dr. Zdeblick had signed a ten-year contract with Medtronic in 1998 that required him to consult with the company for two days every three months, a total of eight days per year, for which he would be paid $400,000. The payments were reportedly stopped in 2004. According to the article, "Dr. Zdeblick, who is a defendant in the lawsuit but who said he was unaware of the accusations against him, said he worked much more than what was required, as many as three or four days a month."

If Dr. Zdeblick's 1993 paper had minor implications, it would not be important to seek the answers. However, this is a paper that is the quintessential definition of an entire specialty, and as a spine surgeon, I need answers.

What baffles me is how the scientific community and the leaders of spine surgery stand by and accept an unfinished study as a reference for all the work that they do. Am I the only surgeon who sets a high bar for the quality of research that we accept? What we do in America permeates to the rest of the world, and the rest of the world is trusting us to do the right thing. Unfortunately, we have failed ourselves and the entire world by not probing and questioning a pivotal piece of medical research.

The Opposing Research

Now I would like to present six prospective, randomized studies that were published in reputable journals. They all say that the addition of pedicle screws to spinal fusion does *not* improve the outcome, and the addition of pedicle screws to spinal fusion does *not* increase the fusion rate, both of which directly contradict Dr. Zdeblick's study.

The first paper, by Thomsen, Christensen, et al., was published in the December 15, 1997, issue of *Spine*. This was a very good study, and it won the 1997 Volvo Award for clinical studies. The Volvo Award was given to studies that were well conducted with a very valued outcome. For this study, a total of 130 patients were randomly selected to receive pedicle screws or to receive the same surgery without implantation of pedicle screws. These patients were followed for two years after the surgery. They achieved 97.7 percent follow-up after two years. This study showed that there was no difference between the two groups in functional outcome and fusion rate. They concluded that the addition of pedicle screws increased operation time, blood loss, and reoperative rate, and they added significant risk of nerve injury. They concluded that there was no justification for the general use of pedicle screws when performing posterior lumbar fusion.

The second paper was published by France, Yaszemski, et al. in the March 15, 1999 issue of *Spine*. They did a prospective randomized study among seventy-one patients. They randomly divided patients into two groups. One group received pedicle screws after lumbar fusion, and the second group did not receive pedicle screws after the completion of lumbar fusion. These patients were also followed for two years. This study showed that there was no difference in reported outcomes between the two groups. They also concluded that there was no benefit of adding pedicle screws in lumbar fusions.

The third study was published in the June 1, 2002, issue of *Spine* by Fritzell, Hägg, et al. This was again a prospective, randomized clinical study, this time with a five-year follow-up. They found the reoperation rate in the group that received pedicle screws was 25 percent as opposed to 14 percent for patients that did not receive pedicle screws. They concluded that there was no difference in outcome between the patients who received pedicle screws and the patients who did not receive pedicle screws. They concluded that pedicle screw implantation increased the reoperation rate.

The fourth paper was published in the June 15, 2002, issue of *Spine* by Christensen, Hansen, Laursen, and Thomsen. The goal was to obtain functional outcomes in patients suffering from severe low back pain treated by posterolateral spinal fusion with or without pedicle screw instrumentation. This study showed no correlation between functional outcome and that the use of instrument pedicle screws did not influence lumbar spinal alignment.

The fifth paper was published in *Journal of Spinal Disorders & Techniques* in its June 2002 issue by Korsgaard, Christensen, et al. This was a prospective, randomized study, multicenter, with a two-year follow-up. They divided patients into three categories, and they also used an independent observer to collect and interpret the data. They concluded that all forms of fusion, with or without instrumentation, improved outcome significantly. However, there was no disadvantage in not using pedicle screws or other instrumentation.

The sixth paper was published by Jäger, Seller, Raab, et al. in *Medical Science* in its July 2003 issue. They looked at thirty-three patients with and without instrumentation. Their conclusions were that the results did not indicate a benefit in outcome from adding pedicle screws in elective lumbar fusions.

I need to state that I am not a keyboard warrior, and I am not just writing this book to complain about the state of spine surgery. I am actually fighting in the trenches. When I spoke to one of the professors at St. Louis University and expressed my concern about the literature and pedicle screws, he said that these papers were old. My answer was that there is no expiration date on these studies.

I walked into my office about six months after that conversation, and I had the latest copy of *Spine* on my desk from December 1, 2018. The lead article, by William Abdu and Olivia Sacks, caught my eye. This was a very anticipated study. It was a randomized study that had an eight-year follow-up with patients who had nonoperative treatment compared to operative treatment. For the operative treatment, they compared people who received pedicle screws to people who did not receive pedicle screws. This was a very important article. This study showed that people who underwent surgery had a much better outcome after eight years of follow-up as opposed to not having the surgery.

The literature to this point is consistent and shows that the surgeries we do as spine surgeons improve the quality of our patients' lives. However, in this 2018 study, the authors observed that the outcome did not matter whether pedicle screws were added to spinal fusion or not. Two decades have gone by since the first of these studies, and everything is the same. It feels like we have not gained anything in the world of spine surgery whatsoever, in spite of the innovations that have come and gone.

The Problem for Spine Surgery

The studies that I presented here so far are well known to leaders of spine surgery. Most academics have the same attitude that they share. "We know that we have not been able to show with research that pedicle screws work, but we will in the future." They have no further explanation.

My message to these surgeons and academics in writing this book is that so far, we have clearly shown by research that pedicle screws do not work. Every time we fail to show that these screws work, we are actually showing that these screws don't work. The burden of proof is on us as surgeons. We are implanting these devices in our patients. It is our duty to show we are doing the right thing by them. For every study that might show pedicle screws do not work, we should have two studies showing that they do – if that were really the case. In the field of medicine, you cannot just break even. So far, however, the evidence against screws is overwhelming. This is the very definition of insanity—we are doing the same experiment over and over and hoping that in the future one will have a different outcome.

The motion of the spinal bone is rotational. We have asked screws to stop rotational motion, which the screw is not made for. We also tell the screw to do that using spongy bone, which is weak. When the results come back that it does not work, we don't want to believe the results.

146

The problem that spine surgery is facing is much deeper. We have used general orthopedic long-bone fracture principles to treat spine conditions. That's wrong. We have to study and develop principles specific to the spine and use those principles to invent new devices and treat spinal conditions. The analogy would be similar to Newtonian and quantum physics. If you want to build a house, you can do that using Newtonian physics. However, if you try to study light and build lasers, you have to use totally different principles from quantum physics.

Spine surgery from the beginning has been derailed by going in the wrong direction. Now we have to set the world of spine surgery back on the right course.

I'd like to finish this chapter with another story that illustrates what I've been up against for years. I was attending a major spine conference in 2016. During an open discussion, I got up and expressed my dissatisfaction with pedicle screws. I was not confrontational in any way; I merely gave my opinion that the screws did more harm than good. After I said my piece, I sat down, and no one said anything. Twenty minutes later, during a break, I was getting coffee and started talking with one of the other surgeons. He then introduced me to another gentleman sitting behind us.

The first doctor said to the second, "Dr. Aslie doesn't like pedicle screws." The second one said, "Oh, you're the guy that made those comments. Well, I have to say everyone is entitled to his opinion, but needless to say you are very wrong."

I explained to them both that it's not about me, it's about the research. The research says that the screws don't work.

The second surgeon introduced himself and said, "I did major research into this subject, and the papers I coauthored were all about my patients."

I won't mention any of the names, but I will say that he was well-known. As it happened, I was holding the journals with all six of the articles that supported my position. The surgeon I was talking to was a coauthor on one of the papers I had in my hands. I pulled it out and he said, "Yes, that's me!"

I said, "Okay, let's read your article," and I started to read him a section of his own journal article, word for word. The last line of the article said that pedicle screws do not increase fusion rates and should not be used routinely.

You might think that would have confirmed my argument, but it didn't. The surgeon focused on his paper, stroked his chin, and finally said, "No way. That is wrong." And then he walked away.

To anyone who might ask me why haven't I presented my concerns to leaders in the field, the answer is, I have. I have chased them down, I have confronted them, I have pleaded with them. There was one surgeon at a cervical spine research society meeting who I begged to give me five minutes. He said no. He made me feel like I was a panhandler.

The responses I have received from leaders in the field, even the ones who have coauthored papers that go against the use of pedicle screws, have been deafening silence. It defies logic. I have tried everything, and so here we are.

CHAPTER SIX

~

My Journey

I t's easy to write off people who have no credentials or experience and to discredit others for being disreputable or having axes to grind. I don't fit into either category, which readers of this book will understand when they hear my story. I consider myself the least likely person to discover an apparent conspiracy by medical device companies or to stir up controversy for personal gain or benefit. If I had become a spine surgeon and found that the information and techniques I learned worked well all the time, as with orthopedic surgeons who set broken arms and legs, no doubt I would have had an uneventful but successful career taking care of patients and earning a good living in the process. I never sought to disagree or quarrel with colleagues, and I always tell young surgeons to never pick fights with colleagues—you never know when you might need them. I never tried to do anything other than practice medicine with the very highest levels of integrity, honesty, and principle. I did not go looking for trouble, but when I discovered that medical device companies had pushed spine surgery into a dead end and turned the field into what I believe is the biggest scam in medicine, I could not stay silent. I value self-respect far more than money.

One of the most important things to note when reading a scientific paper is who the author is. You need to know their credentials, their activities, and most of all, their character. It was a difficult decision to include a chapter about my life, but I decided that for readers to truly understand how I uncovered the scheme of device-making companies, I had to tell my story. I am not trying to brag, by any means. I believe one of the most important accomplishments in life is to have friends that care about you. Bragging is a very good way of making yourself lonely. When I won the Innovations Showcase at the Congress of Neurological Surgeons in 2015, which is really a lifetime achievement, the only person I told was my wife. I had to tell her because she was getting nervous about how much money I was spending on my project.

Early Life

I was born in a small town in Iran. After my mother and father divorced, I moved to Tehran with my mother and sister. My father was a physician and a city coroner. I was extremely close to my father even though my parents were divorced. When I was eight years old, I watched my father perform an autopsy through a cracked-open door. I also used to attend investigations with him, and I attended an autopsy with my father at the age of nine. From a very young age, I planned to become a doctor. I did not think of myself doing anything else because I was so close to my father. I wanted to go to the same prep school that my father attended in Tehran and to attend Tehran University for medical school.

When I was fourteen years old, the revolution happened in Iran, and there was a change in government. The Shah of Iran, the country's monarch, was overthrown and replaced by the Islamic Republic. Soon after, when I was fifteen, the Iran–Iraq War started. This was a very bloody war, and about half a million people died with really no change by the time it ended in 1988.

I was an excellent student at Alborz High School, the prep school that my father attended and the best high school in Iran. When I was seventeen years old, my family realized a very serious problem: once I turned eighteen, I would be required to serve in the military and be sent to fight in the Iran–Iraq War. There was a high likelihood of being killed. Since all I wanted was to become a doctor, I needed to escape from the country.

I could almost write two books about my adventures of escaping from Iran, but I will only mention the essential parts. The area I crossed was the northwestern part of Iran called Azerbaijan, which borders Turkey and Russia. It is a mountainous region, and the majority of the villages are of Kurdish ethnicity. At that time, in addition to the ongoing war with Iraq, there was an internal conflict with the Kurdish people seeking independence. Kurdish people are some of the nicest people I have ever met in the world. They are very hardworking and honest. Unfortunately, they are spread out over four countries: Turkey, Syria, Iraq, and Iran. Because they are minorities in each country, they are constantly mistreated by these central governments. I had no choice but to escape through an active war zone.

The war I was trying to avoid involved three powers: the Kurdish militia, the Iranian Army, and the Revolutionary Guards. The Kurdish militia was fighting for independence and was mostly comprised of local villagers. The next two powers were part of Iranian government forces. Right after the revolution, the Shah's Army was dismantled, and a lot of the generals and high-ranking officers were jailed. However, as the war with Iraq started and the uprising in the Kurdish region intensified, the Islamic government realized they needed pilots and highly skilled officers to operate the heavy weaponry. Many were released from jail and given their posts back. Therefore, the second group, the Iranian Army, was the remnant of the Shah's Army and comprised of the Shah's officers. The third group was called the Revolutionary Guards. This was a militia and religious faction that was part of the government, the Mujahideen militia, who had no formal training in war. Most of their weapons were light and portable, so they relied on the regular army for support with heavy weaponry.

The mentality of the Iranian Army, as remnants from the Shah's time, was that Iranian people were Iranian citizens, and they did not want to go fight them. Such was the beauty of Iran under the Shah. Iran was composed of many ethnic groups and was very diverse. We were all Iranians, and nobody cared about ethnicity. No one ever asked somebody what their ethnicity was simply because they did not care. The group I feared most were the Revolutionary Guards because they did care about ethnicity, and they expected strict adherence to their laws and religion. Remaining in Tehran was, for me, not an option; I had to escape.

When I say escape, it does not mean that I was by myself hiking around the mountains. Despite the chaos, there was extreme order. The local villagers organized and formed bands to transport people who were leaving Iran. The escaping people were taken by guides from village to village and eventually crossed the border to Turkey and into a major city, most likely Istanbul. In a war zone, you have to be with a guide. If you are caught by yourself, the assumption would be that you belonged to the other faction, which would mean serious trouble for you. At that time, there was a significant exodus of young men escaping the war to seek higher education in outside countries. It was common for people my age to go through this region, and the local villages were used to it.

However, my situation had some complications. I was supposed to be taken by a guide to a village on the Iranian side that was extremely close to the border. Someone was then supposed to come from across the border and take me to Istanbul. I was eventually taken with guides, and we hiked pretty much from eight in the evening to four in the morning, and we made it to the village on the Iranian side. But the person who was supposed to come and get me at the village did not show up. I found myself stuck on the Iranian side of the border with no clear idea of when or how I might be able to leave.

The village was extremely remote and primitive, with no electricity and no communication with the outside world. That said, the Kurdish villagers were absolutely the best. I became friendly with them and quickly felt at home after only a few days. Their food was amazing, and they were very welcoming.

There were twenty to thirty homes in this village, all made from clay and brick. There was no road coming in from the valley, which made it even more isolated. In spite of this, the people who lived there were very well informed through word of mouth. I enjoyed talking and hanging out with them. I stayed in one of the homes, where I ate breakfast, lunch, and dinner, feeling very much as if I were a part of their family. Looking back after many years, I wish I could go back and thank them. I didn't fully appreciate what they did for me because I was in a very bad situation. I was treated like a member of the family. But it was still a war zone, and the mood was not happy.

Day seven of my stay started just like any other day. But when I got up to walk around, I noticed that there were not many people in the village. I had become friendly with the local militia leaders who were staying in a tent. I walked up to the tent, sat down, and started listening to the Kurdish militia commandos. It turned out that the men and boys of the village had gone on patrol of the valley and the bottom of the hill, something they did routinely. I do not remember anybody using radios; there was no contact with the militia.

As the commandos were talking, we heard some explosions in the distance. The commandos looked at one another with concern. We then heard helicopters getting close. One of the commandos screamed to get out of the tent because they knew it would be a target. We ran into the woods, a tiny area of only twenty square yards with trees that were very tall and skinny. The villagers use these trees to build homes. Another commando ran down the hill and screamed at us to get out, fearing that the trees were also a target. Then he, too, ran off.

At that point, it was just me and two seasoned Kurdish commandoes, each of them with six to eight AK-47 clips around their belly and two yellow grenades hanging from their shoulders. The three of us ran toward a dirt road that was about fifty yards away with a ditch on the other side big enough for only two people. The two men did a commando roll into the ditch. Once there, they looked back at me with an expression that said, "What are you doing standing there, kid?"

I was a seventeen-year-old boy from a prep school who had watched many war movies, but I had absolutely no training. In the movies, soldiers ran, the bullets caught up to them, and they dropped. I decided not to run because I knew the bullets would catch up with me and I would die. It is hard to explain, but before this event, I always thought that if I were ever in a combat situation, I imagined that there would be a lot of things I could possibly do, like finding a weapon to fire back at the enemy. I learned a big lesson that day. I learned not to say what I would do in certain situations. Once you are in a situation without having any training, things are completely different.

I froze. My heart never beat so fast and so strong in my entire life ever again. The commandos must have thought I was either incredibly stupid or incredibly brave for standing out in the open. I looked up and saw the belly of a Cobra helicopter overhead. For five horrifying seconds, the Cobra passed within a few meters and fired its main cannon. After the helicopter made a second pass over the village, the pilot turned away and left.

When the Cobra was well out of sight, the commandos climbed out of the ditch and came toward me; I was unable to speak. As we walked together toward the village, they talked about seeing carnage and bodies. We thought we might have lost at least half of the village, which would have been absolutely devastating. Instead, we found the villagers all alive and the buildings intact. But we also heard women and children in the village crying. Their husbands and sons were still out there, and they feared the worst.

The first or second day that I was at the village, I asked the commandos a lot of questions about their weapons, such as if they had anti-aircraft guns or heavy artillery. Like I said, I had watched plenty of war movies, and I was a very curious seventeen-year-old. The mood of the conversation completely changed at that point, and suddenly I felt that they suspected me of being a spy. They asked the village elder why I was inquiring about the heavy weapons. I started shaking and wondered to myself why I had stupidly asked sensitive questions. I wanted to tell them that I was only curious. The elder shook his head and told them that I was just a kid and not to worry about my questions. I breathed a sigh of relief, and that was the end of it.

Now I made a mistake a second time. I did not see anyone carrying a radio, and we had no clear idea what had happened to the rest of the villagers, so I asked the commando if he had a radio. He gave me a look that I will never forget, and I immediately realized my mistake and cut the conversation extremely short. Lesson learned. In an active war zone, never ask questions or talk about war.

About three hours later, the villagers who were on patrol started trickling back; it was a joyous sight. Apparently, no one got even a scratch on them. The entire village became jubilant and happy now that it was becoming clear everyone was safe—miraculously so.

This was a mountainous area, but there were no large rocks. This part of the mountain was flat with very short grass and no rocks to hide behind. The villagers explained to us that they were actually surprised to see a Huey gunship and a Cobra helicopter patrolling on the hill. They said that the helicopters could have decimated them if they wanted to. Instead, the helicopters signaled with three flashes of their headlights to warn the men on patrol to disperse and run away. The helicopters started firing their machine guns at the bottom of the hill, then at the top of the hill, then launching their rockets toward the opposite hill, but they weren't trying to hit anyone or anything—they were trying to miss. This allowed the pilots to tell the story as they wished when they returned to their base. They had to use the ammunition because there were probably forward observers monitoring what was going on. The villagers understood that the pilots were from the time of the Shah's Army.

If I didn't hear it with my own ears, I would never believe it. It made a significant impact on me. I saw that, even in the middle of a war, humanity is not dead and we can still be civil.

My guide showed up three days after this incident and took me to Istanbul.

Medical School in Ankara, Turkey

I spent almost three years in Turkey as a refugee, where I studied hard and did well academically. I was able to sign up for the university entrance exam, and I got into the best medical school in Turkey, called Hacettepe University, in Ankara.

I was not, however, home free. I had to go through very difficult times to escape from Iran to get to Turkey, and I was a man with no country. I could not go to the Iranian embassy because I had escaped, and I did not have a passport from any other country. I had a very unpredictable future as a refugee in Turkey. Since I was able to attend medical school, though, I was in heaven. All my life, I had dreamt of going to medical school, and there I was. I was extremely enthusiastic and walking on clouds.

When I started my anatomy class, I was excited to work on cadavers. This was a big moment for me because as a child I had heard stories from my father about his time in medical school and his time studying anatomy with cadavers.

The class of about 150 was divided into four groups. Each group had an assigned associate professor; my group had Mr. Erdogan (not his real name). This Mr. Erdogan seemed to be a very unhappy character. It almost seemed like he never smiled or laughed in his life. He was very rough. I never saw him talking to anyone outside of work. The associate professors would do the dissections the night before, and the next day the parts we were studying were already labeled for us so that we could study anatomy in the cadaver lab. Even though that was important to me, I wanted to actually be part of the dissection because I eventually wanted to become a surgeon. I asked if I could help the associate professors on the other teams. I was informed that I needed to stick to my own team.

One afternoon around five thirty, I showed up to the lab, and I saw that Mr. Erdogan was dissecting the cadaver. I approached him slowly, and I started shaking as I got close. I do not believe he even looked at me for a few minutes. I asked him very politely if there was any way that I could help him. He said that he did not need any help. I told him that I just wanted the chance to show him that I could help him, but he would not budge. This conversation went back and forth for a few minutes. I was begging him to let me help him, and he became more and more upset. At some point, he asked me to leave as he did not need any help, and I would need to wait to see everything the following day.

At this point, I was not shaking anymore, and I had a surge of power through me like lightning. I remember pointing to the ground and telling him that I would not leave the spot unless he let me help him. At that moment, I saw his expression change. I did not know what he was going to do next, but I was not going to leave under any circumstances. He finally said, "Fine, come and help me with this part." We started working together after that and actually hit it off. He was not the horrible man that I was led to believe. His concerns were very legitimate, and we worked well together. He may not have been the friendliest man, but I learned quite a bit from him, and that was all I cared about.

About three months later, the time came for our final exam. I was studying in the anatomy lab and looking at a cadaver. The associate professors were talking at the table about six to ten feet away from me, and I could hear them clearly. One of the associate professors asked

Mr. Erdogan about his group of students. Mr. Erdogan said he was not so sure about the Turkish students, but the Iranian students were very smart and were going to do great. Hearing him say that put a smile on my face, and I was proud of what I had accomplished. We took the final exam, and our group of Iranian students all did very well.

One year went by, and I was sitting having lunch in a group with my classmates and three Iranian upperclassmen. Out of the blue, Mr. Erdogan crossed in front of us on his way to the cafeteria. The upperclassmen acted like they wanted to avoid eye contact with him. They pointed and said this guy is so horrible and made it clear that he hated Iranians. My classmates looked at each other in disbelief. We started saying that it was not true and that he loved us. It immediately hit me that it was not true that he hated Iranians. The upperclassmen were just not very good students.

This simple comment of unjustly labeling Mr. Erdogan had a very profound effect on me and actually shaped my future. I thought about this interaction long and hard for many years. I thought if I had this conversation with the upperclassmen before my interaction with Mr. Erdogan, it would have been completely different. Throughout my time with Mr. Erdogan, it never even remotely crossed my mind that he might treat me differently or like me differently because I was a foreigner. However, it might have crossed my mind after hearing the comments from the upperclassmen, and that would have been detrimental to the development of my relationship with him. I had developed mutual respect with Mr. Erdogan. That interaction always stayed in my mind. From that, I learned not to take the opinions of others at face value. They could be wrong. They could be biased. They could be misinformed. I needed to think for myself, and from then on, I did.

Moving to America

After four years, I came to the United States as an immigrant. When I came to America, I promised myself that I would never allow myself to be treated differently because I am Iranian. I worked hard, and I listened to criticism. If I was criticized, I took responsibility for it. My reaction was that yes, you are right, and I have to do better. I truly believe this attitude has had a lot to do with my success in my academic career and my private practice. I am sure I have bumped into people that were not very friendly, but it never crossed my mind that I was treated differently because I was a foreigner. Even if I did come across angry people, my attitude was that it was absolutely not my problem, and it never bothered me.

My advice to young people is that I have never seen hard work go to waste. The second thing I tell them is that everyone will love you if you work hard. I always tell young people that listening to criticism is the only way you can get better, and you have to get better. There is always room for improvement. The best advice I've heard comes from the pro football player Tom Brady. He said, "See, there are a lot of guys who are all talk. They say they want to work harder and be the best, but they never pay the price." That is how I have been in my practice and in my research and development. My attitude is that we can always do better and work harder. We cannot be satisfied with what we have in hand when it comes to patient care.

This is one of the biggest issues I have when I debate spine surgeons that I meet in conferences. This includes so-called leaders of the field. When I point to the shortcomings of pedicle screws and the literature, 80 percent of the surgeons have the exact same response. Their response is that their patients are doing great, and they do not see any problem with the use of pedicle screws in their practice. The great majority of surgeons that I debate and present with my case are very happy with where they are in their practice. I try to enlighten them. I tell them that there are two layers that make it unacceptable to be happy with the way things are. One is that the research and the publications do not say that the patients are not doing well. The published papers say that spine surgery is generally successful in alleviating pain, and patients do well getting the surgery as opposed to not getting the surgery. However, the research also says that the addition of the pedicle screws does not add any benefit to the outcome of the surgery. That means that a cheap surgery is just as good as a very expensive surgery.

As surgeons, we can never be satisfied with the way our practice stands. We are talking about patient care and health. If there is even one unsatisfied patient in my practice, I am not satisfied. As Tom Brady says, it does not matter how good you are or how many Superbowl wins you have; there is always room for improvement. That is how a spine surgeon should think. The moment you are happy with the way things are done, that is the moment you stop progressing. I believe our patients deserve better.

It seems that sort of attitude cannot be learned; you have to be born with it. Maybe that is one of the reasons that I am the one who understands the apparent conspiracy and exposes the instrument companies who have forcefully applied and maintained the status quo in the world of spine surgery. To them, it is about making the most money possible; to me, it is about doing the right thing for patients.

I transferred my two years of medical school in Turkey to University of California, Berkeley, where I studied physiology and genetics as an undergraduate. I entered Berkeley as a junior. Being a true immigrant, my mother and I were very poor when I arrived in the United States, and we lived in the same room. It is very difficult to describe the feeling I had when I came to the United States. I am not sure if it is a feeling that everybody gets, but I felt deeply grateful about being able to get a green card and come to the United States to continue my education.

America is the greatest country in the world and a world leader. I knew of many talented, smart friends that were left in Iran. I felt I was representing them and had a sense of responsibility. I also felt chosen to have this privilege. It was important not to let the opportunity go to waste. When I came to America, I felt it was not just about my life, but about representing a group of people. This was not necessarily just the

Iranian friends and family that I had left in Iran, but the entire community that I lived in. I got to work. I focused on studying and nothing else.

When I first arrived, my mother wanted me to get a job, but I refused. I told her that my job was to study. My sister was angry with my mother for not making me get a job, so my mom was under pressure from her. I continued to refuse to get a job, and my mother was struggling with what to do about me. My mother told me that things are different in America and here you must go to school and work at the same time. She told me that she did not have the financial means to support me completely, so I would need to chip in.

One night her feelings changed. She woke up at 3:00 a.m. to use the bathroom and saw the kitchen light was on. She saw me studying with three books in front of me. She apparently decided that it would be best for me to focus on studying even if we had to eat cardboard. I felt it was my responsibility to focus on nothing but studying. I did not care about partying. I wanted to date and have a social life, but I shelved that during that part of my life because I had more important things to accomplish.

I could not have achieved what I have if I did not have family support, especially to that extent. I am not talking about monetary support—monetary support is probably the least important thing. When I was applying to medical school, I was naïve, and I had to learn my lessons, in particular humility. Yes, you have to have self-confidence, but you always have to be ready for adversity. In my life, every time I had adversity, I got up swinging and ended up in a better place. I had many friends during college and medical school who had to do this by themselves without family support. I truly believe if they had the support that I had, they would have achieved far greater academic success.

For example, when I was applying to medical school after Berkeley, I was inexperienced and stupid in terms of applications and interviews. My sister showed me her wisdom, and I am truly grateful to her for buying me a plane ticket and talking me into going for an interview in New York. This had a significant impact on my life. I would like to apologize to my sister for giving her such a hard time, but I ended up listening to what she wanted me to do.

Medical School at New York Medical College

There is not really much that I can say about my experience in medical school because all I did was study and study some more. I made some friends that I continue to have to this day. On a typical day, I would wake up at 7:00 a.m. and be out of the house by 7:30. I would get to school, and classes would start by 8:00 then continue until about 2:00. By three p.m., I would be back home to relax so that by four I would be asleep and then wake up around six thirty or seven. When I got up, I would fix myself dinner then study from 8:00 p.m. until 4:00 a.m. Then I would sleep again and wake up at 7:00 a.m. to repeat the process all over again. I divided my sleep time into two periods of three hours, which was the most efficient way of using my time. On the weekends, I caught up on my sleep, and sometimes I did not wake up until noon on Saturday. I would also wake up around noon on Sunday, then start studying again.

With nothing else to do but study, I was able to rank number one in my class during the first two years, which were the academic years. The third and fourth years of medical school were clinical rotations, and I was able to be quite successful. I received high honors in all my surgical rotations.

By the end of my third year, I was dead set on becoming a cardiac surgeon. I was attracted to cardiac surgery because it was highly prestigious and attracted the best of the best. I also spent some time in the cardiac unit and was amazed that cardiac surgeons were able to stop the heart, perform surgery, restart the heart, and literally bring the patient back to life. I truly believed that cardiac surgeons were absolutely the best doctors. My first choice was a program called East Bay Surgery Residency Program, and my plan was a ten-year path to becoming a cardiac surgeon.

Those plans were completely derailed. At the end of my internship year, medical device companies came out with stents. A stent is a spring that is placed into the coronaries to keep them open. Before stents, the minimally invasive procedure was angioplasty, which is the placement of a balloon into the coronary artery to blow it up and open the blockage. One of the problems with angioplasty is the reclosure of the coronary artery. However, with the invention of the stent, the coronary would stay open, and there was no need for open-heart surgery, and the demand for cardiac surgeons was likely to drop precipitously.

Once stents came onto the market, I had to think fast. I was on a ten-year path of grueling study to do one surgery very well: cardiac bypass surgery. Now I could see the minimally invasive alternatives to open-heart surgery were becoming available, and I thought the technology favored invasive cardiology as opposed to open-heart surgery. Open-heart surgery was a dying field, and minimally invasive cardiology was much more supported by technology.

That is why I decided to switch my residency. It turned out to be the correct move. Within the past two decades, cardiac surgery has played less and less of a role in managing coronary artery disease. Noninvasive cardiology can do procedures that we could not dream of in the past. With minimally invasive techniques, cardiologists can manage more and more severe conditions. Within the past five years, I have met two cardiothoracic surgeons who could not find jobs in their specialty.

Changing residencies is extremely difficult, especially if you have to change your residency to something that is even more popular. Through great persistence, I was able to switch my residency and enter orthopedic surgery. I started a residency program at St. Vincent's Hospital in Greenwich Village in New York. I truly had memorable years studying there.

During that time, I developed a significant interest in spine surgery, and I became very close with my professors and my chairman, who was a world-renowned scoliosis surgeon. After completing my residency in orthopedic surgery at St. Vincent's, I was able to secure a fellowship in spine surgery at Beth Israel Hospital in Boston under the supervision of one of the forefathers of spine surgery. This program was part of Harvard Medical School.

Starting My Practice

After completion of my fellowship, I started looking for a job. Due to the fact that my family was living in the Bay Area, I was looking for jobs in Northern California. At the time, the only position that was available in Northern California that I could find was a position with a small medical group called Sutter North in Yuba City, California. So, I started my practice in Yuba City, California, as part of Sutter North Medical Group. After two years, I branched off and went into private practice as a solo practitioner in spine surgery.

When I went to Yuba City, I planned to stay for just two years to get my board certification, then leave for a more cosmopolitan city, such as San Francisco or Los Angeles. However, after two years, I felt at home and had grown to like the community. By 2005, I was board certified. By 2007, I was five years into my private practice and doing very well. I was actually in a very good spot. I was in private practice by myself, I had not been involved in any sort of lawsuit or had any problems with my surgeries, and I had developed a good, solid reputation in the region. All my friends and family were in the Bay Area, and I traveled to see them almost every weekend. My life was good and solid. Six years into my practice, I had established myself in the community, I loved my patients and referring physicians, and my patients loved me.

When I got my job in the small town of Yuba City, I really did not have any aspirations to become a world-renowned surgeon or become famous whatsoever. I was quite satisfied with my job and with my situation in private practice. However, there was one problem in the back of my mind. I realized there was a stigma attached to practicing in a small town. I felt that patients and referring physicians once in a while would not value me as a very reliable and solid authority, because who has heard of Yuba City? Sometimes I had the feeling that the word on the street was that if you wanted to get a solid consultation or see a surgeon that really knows what they are doing, you had to go to a bigger city like Sacramento or preferably San Francisco.

It's probably true in every profession that the bigger the city you practice in, the more solid your foundation and truer your opinions. For example, if you are practicing in a small town like Yuba City, you are not considered as good as the doctors practicing in Sacramento, and if you are practicing in Sacramento, you are not as good as some of the doctors who practice in San Francisco, and if you are practicing in San Francisco, you might not be as good as some of the doctors who are practicing in New York City, and so on.

Sometimes I could ignore it, but other times it really bothered me quite a bit. After all, I had gone to Berkeley, competed with the best, and did very well. This was true for my boards, my MCAT scores, GPAs, etc. I also had my training at Harvard University. I really did not think of myself as less worthy than the surgeons who were practicing at UC Davis or UCSF. I felt quite capable and confident. Sometimes I thought practicing in a small town by myself actually gave me more confidence. I know that most of the surgeons who join big practices will continue for a while as if they are training in school. They start with the easier cases under supervision or a mentor in the big practice and, as they go along, they are able to branch out and take on more complex cases. However, I started my practice with absolutely no supervision or backup.

The most difficult surgery I have done to this day was the very first surgery I did in my entire career. This was a very difficult patient, a woman with severe spinal stenosis in the lumbar spine with cauda equina syndrome. She had been sent to me by a neurosurgeon. When that patient showed up at my office, she had difficulty with bowel and bladder function, and so I had to take her to surgery right away. I had to do a couple of original tricks to complete the surgery, which I did entirely by myself with the help of a scrub nurse.

At some point in the middle of the surgery, I was very scared. To be honest, I doubted myself. But I was able to collect my thoughts and come up with a method of problem-solving, and I was able to complete the surgery with great results. It was not difficult just because it was my first surgery; even if that factor is taken out, it is still the most difficult surgery I have done in my entire twenty years of practice due to the severity of the pathology. I completed the surgery with the confidence that I could do anything. I do not recommend going that route because the surgery really shook me. But it did turn out well for me, and it paved a path for the future of my career.

The Comment That Changed My Life

From the get-go, I was doing complex cases without help, and I quickly developed self-confidence in my work. The fact that I was a spine surgeon in a small town did not bother me, but a comment made by a patient or referring physician might occasionally bother me. Then there was one rude comment by a surgeon from San Francisco that changed the entire course of my life.

I had a patient who had severe disc damage and herniation at the level of L3-4 and L5-S1. That means the patient had two very badly damaged discs with one very healthy disc in the middle. This was a workers' compensation patient, which meant that neither the patient nor I had a say in terms of overall management. This patient was also sent by workers' compensation to a surgeon in San Francisco for a second opinion. For a period of four months, this patient went back and forth between me and the surgeon in San Francisco.

Once the patient completed the entire course of nonoperative care, including multiple steroid injections and multiple sessions of physical rehab, he was still very symptomatic with severe lower back pain. The time had come, and the patient decided to proceed with surgery. My recommendation for the patient was to have a two-level fusion at the level of L3-4 and L5-S1, leaving the disc at the level of L4-5 alone. I had thought about this case for many months and had decided that I could not bring myself to fuse the disc in the middle because it was perfectly fine.

The surgeon in San Francisco recommended a three-level fusion, which included the healthy disc at the level of L4-5. His rationale was that the L4-5 disc would be between the two fused levels and would be under a tremendous amount of stress, which would lead to another surgery in the future to fuse that disc. Therefore, he wanted to include it in the fusion.

The patient returned to inform me what the surgeon in San Francisco had planned. I explained to the patient that I totally understood where the surgeon was coming from, and I did not disagree with him. I told the patient that it might be the best way to go. However, as a spine surgeon, I simply could not bring myself to fuse a disc that was perfectly normal just because it might go bad in the future. I told the patient that if another surgery was required to fuse the L4-5 disc in the future, so be it, but I did not recommend including that disc in the fusion. I would fuse the L3-4 and the L5-S1 discs separately. I also explained to the patient that a three-level fusion from L3 to S1 would put extra pressure on the L2-3 disc space, and the L2-3 disc level could go bad faster.

The patient went back to San Francisco, and the next time he saw me, he mentioned a comment the surgeon in San Francisco had made, word for word. Apparently, the surgeon in San Francisco said to the patient, "You either get your surgery done in Yuba City, or you get it done right."

That comment hurt me quite a bit. It put a knife right where I felt vulnerable. After all my academic achievements, I felt that practicing in a small town might not be the glory I deserved. I had thought about this topic in the past and had come to the conclusion that it does not matter where you practice. You are either taking care of patients in a large city or taking care of patients in a small town, and it does not matter. This comment opened up this wound. However, I was hurt for only about one month.

I am a person who does not normally get upset, and I like to turn negative energy into positive energy. I made a conscious decision. I decided that the only way to fight this feeling and put this argument to rest was to invent the most important device in the world of spine surgery. That way, I could show the world that even though I practice in a small town, I am as good as anybody else. That is how everything changed for me.

I truly believe that every one of us has a gift; it is left for us to find out what that gift is. I've discovered that mine is being able to visualize which medical procedures are possible and which are not. Between 2004 and 2010, there was a significant boom in the world of spine surgery in terms of new devices and techniques. One company invented a new technique called XLIF. In this surgery, the surgeon could approach the spine from the side of the patient, which made it minimally invasive. Representatives of the company visited all the surgeons in the Sacramento area, and all of them expressed great concern about the potential dangers. They flat-out refused to do the surgery. When I was presented with the surgery, I immediately recognized its potential. I went through the training program and, a week later, I had a patient on the schedule. It turned out that I was the first spine surgeon, at least in Northern California, to perform the surgery. Now, more than a decade later, XLIF surgery is considered the standard of care, and there is a requirement that spine trainees must learn it.

The converse also happened. Around the late 2000s, a new surgery became available: lumbar disc replacement surgery. In that surgery on the lumbar spine, instead of fusing two vertebrae after removing the disc, the surgeon places a prosthesis that allows motion. I remember when I went for training, and we were bussed to the facility. The sight was unbelievable. Lines of buses, each carrying thirty surgeons, were lined up around the training center. They were booked months in advance, such was the enthusiasm for the procedure. I remember the instructor telling us that once we learned the surgery, we would never want to do any other. When I returned from training, I heard and noticed other surgeons in town doing tons of lumbar disc replacements. I once overheard a patient say that another surgeon in the area had explained to him that fusion surgery is like "Volkswagen surgery, and disc replacement is like Bentley surgery." In the hospital, I could see on the board that my colleagues were doing multiple lumbar disc replacements per day.

Patients came to see me and demanded that I do disc replacement surgery, but I refused. As I've mentioned repeatedly in this book, the first step in any treatment is to understand the biomechanics of the spine. The main function of the lumbar spine is to support the entire trunk. Anatomy has a lot to do with it. I always think about what-ifs: what if my surgery fails, or what if a patient might need future surgery? What can I do now that will keep the patient from needing dangerous surgery in the future? It turns out that if disc replacement fails, the patient would be in a world of trouble. There were reported deaths during the removal of disc prosthesis. This is because large veins in the abdomen scar down after surgery, and it is extremely dangerous to move them out of the way to get to the prosthesis.

I held off doing any lumbar disc replacements, even though many patients demanded them. I stood my ground. I lost some patients who got their wish by going to other spine surgeons in town, but I did not compromise my principles.

Then the horrible results started pouring in: worsening pain, device failure, and death while attempting to remove the prosthesis. Now a decade later, disc replacement in the lumbar spine is dead, although some companies are trying to bring it back again. It is such a bad idea. I just cannot even imagine the path of destruction this surgery has left behind, the true scope of which will become apparent decades from now. I knew the moment I saw the device that it was destined to fail.

That is my gift. Five years into my practice, I realized that I could look at a device, any orthopedic device, and tell you within minutes if it would work. My father was a physician, but the rest of my family are all engineers, including a great-uncle, uncles, and cousins. My sister is a mechanical engineer working in Silicon Valley. She was the only female in her class. My mother studied math at the University of Tehran and taught math in high school. She was the only female in her class. My fifth-grade daughter scored in the top 99th percentile in the country in the standardized math test. I am not trying to brag, but I think math and engineering are in my blood. I may be deficient in many other qualities, including my organizational skills, but my understanding of biomechanics is innate and infallible. I somehow landed in a job that I was born to do.

Innovating to Solve Problems

It sounds unlikely that someone can just say they are going to invent the most important device in their field, but that is exactly what was in my head. First, I had to identify the most important issue in the world of spine surgery. It was obvious to me at the beginning of my practice that the aging population was increasing in numbers with the baby boomers and, as a group, they faced a significant challenge for spine surgeons. As we age, our bone quality gets pretty bad. The pedicle screw is inserted into the middle of the vertebrae, which is a spongy bone. As I mentioned earlier, the vertebrae are composed of two types of bone. One is the outer shell that we call cortical bone, which is a solid bone. The other is the inside bone, which is spongy bone. We know that the inside bone where the pedicle screws get their purchase is significantly weakened with aging.

It is very well known in the world of spine surgery that anybody above the age of fifty faces weakening spongy bone in the middle of the vertebrae. I explained the anatomy of the vertebrae in Chapter One. The lamina, one of the strongest bones in the body, is the roof of the spinal canal when the patient is lying face down, and it is a purely cortical bone. Therefore, I knew that the aging population was posing a significant challenge to the world of spine surgery.

A lecture I attended by a surgeon in Seattle influenced me greatly. He explained how badly the aging population suffers from this cancellous bone almost dissolving inside of the vertebrae, causing significant problems with the surgery. The pedicle screws frequently loosen or back out, requiring multiple repeated surgeries. I was impressed by that lecture, and I set a goal to solve that problem.

Inventing a device with an anchor that would work better than a pedicle screw became priority number one for me. I started reviewing the literature in detail. I found out that for the last four decades, there was a significant amount of research and a body of work trying to address this very issue. There have been multiple approaches to try to improve the pullout strength of the pedicle screws in the weak cancellous bone of elderly vertebrae, such as adding bone chips to the hole before insertion of the screw, then adding the screw. One of the ways was to actually shoot glue into the hole before inserting the screw, which we call *cement augmentation*. Another way was to change the design of the screw.

There were all sorts of attempts made to change the pitch of the screw to try to optimize the cancellous bone. Screws that expanded were inserted into vertebrae, and a rod was inserted into the core of the screw, causing it to open up like a flower and increase the purchase. Of course, there were some screws that were fenestrated. The surgeon was able to insert the screw, then shoot glue through the core of the screw, which came out through the holes on the sides of the screw and turned into spikes of cement that increased the pullout strength. Some techniques added a wire that went under the lamina, came around the head of the screw, and was twisted by the surgeon so the screw was augmented by a sublaminar wire holding onto the lamina.

There had been an extensive amount of research and work done to try to address the same problem that I was trying to fix. One approach I could make was to find another trick that maybe no one else had thought of to change the grip of the screw. Another possible approach was to forget about the screw and develop a new device that would work completely differently than the screw. I decided that it seemed like everything that could be thought of had already been tried with the screw, and it had not worked. I needed to take the road that no one had ever ventured down and come up with a brand-new device.

To start my project, I had to come up with two important facts. One was that I wanted to go in a different direction. My thinking was that if the bone in the elderly population gets so weak that it does not react well to metal, then maybe we have to put a material between the osteoporotic bone and the metal. This material should be able to hold on to the metal better than bone and likewise can hold on to bone better than metal. We are talking about an intermediary material that needs to be applied. In addition, this device has to hold on to the part of the vertebrae that is the strongest.

I always tell people that I just do not understand the concept of the pedicle screw. A pedicle screw gets inserted into the vertebrae and uses weak cancellous bone for an anchor. That is the problem from the get-go. You always learn that a chain is only as strong as its weakest link. So even if you have a great device that can do great things, if you put it into junky bone, the whole construct is junk. We need to hold on to a part of the vertebrae that is strongest. After a lot of anatomical studies, I decided that the lamina is that part.

Lamina is the part of the vertebrae that all the forces from the paraspinal muscles converge into. This force is transferred through the lamina, into the pedicles, then into the back of the vertebral wall. That is actually how muscles can move the spine in different positions throughout the three-dimensional space. The analogy I make is that if you want to lift up a suitcase, you do not grab it from the corners and you do not shish-kabob it. You hold it by its handle. The spinous vertebrae do have a handle: the lamina. The lamina actually was used as the original anchor for hooks and wires before the introduction of pedicle screws. However, those early devices were not good devices.

When I worked in Yuba City, I lived in Roseville, California. I had to travel back and forth on Highway 65 up to three times a day when I was covering the emergency room. One of the things I constantly saw on that trip were big rigs carrying large loads on their trailers. I observed that the trucks used Kevlar straps to tie down the weight, not metal chains or stainless steel cables. I looked at those trucks and thought that my answer must be something flexible rather than a rigid screw. I decided that I would place an intermediary material between bone and metal, and use lamina as the point of anchor. In a flash, I realized that the answer was to find a material like Kevlar that could be implanted in the human body and last a lifetime.

I got to work. I hired two bioengineers who were experienced in developing spinal implants and set up a lab in Santa Cruz, California. It came in handy that I was an instrument-rated pilot, as I was able to see my patients in the morning in Sacramento and fly to Santa Cruz later in the day to meet with my engineers. For almost four years, I made that commute once every two to three weeks and, in the end, we came up with a working prototype.

I spent just shy of $1 million of my own money on this project over four years; the device is explained in detail in Chapter Eight. The device, which I call a "laminar plating system," is a flat, contoured plate that sits over the laminae and uses a strap that goes around the laminae to secure itself. Therefore, it uses solid cortical bone as opposed to cancellous bone as the anchor. The engineers that I hired and the lab that we set up were world class, and we created publishable data. We did everything to the highest professional standards and to the letter of the book as established by the FDA.

It is simple to build something complex that is supposed to do a complex job, but it is extremely complex to build something simple that does a complex job. There were five or six major steps we had to surpass to make a laminar device for rigid fixation feasible. The device had to achieve immobilization of spinal vertebra—a very complex bone—in a simple manner. It also needed to be placed using a simple procedure and had to be safe for placement in a patient. From personal experience, I knew that if I made a device that worked well in the laboratory, but placement would cause headaches for the surgeon, the device would not be successful.

When I was developing my device, I hit a problem which I cannot disclose but it caused me to go back and study pedicle screws in much more detail. Once I did that, I realized that pedicle screws and the tulip suffered from the same issue, which no one was aware of. I call it "the wolverine phenomenon," which I will discuss in detail in the next chapter.

My knowledge of spine biomechanics increased exponentially as I researched the literature, looking for ways to make a superior device. My studies reinforced my view that the current way of instrumentation in the cervical spine is just barbaric. Each time I do a posterior cervical surgery, I feel guilty as a surgeon. To place our instruments (lateral mass screws), we have to scrape the muscle off the cervical spine all the way from edge to edge. The dissection itself completely destroys the paraspinal muscles. This causes significant pain and discomfort after the surgery. The question is, why do we do this type of surgery at all? We are essentially replacing a sharp, stabbing pain that is absolutely unbearable with a dull, achy pain that can be managed, but we aren't eliminating the pain. One of the benefits of the device I invented is that it is placed in the center of the lamina, which avoids severe dissection laterally.

I took early prototypes to surgical conferences and asked medical colleagues for feedback. Nearly all surgeons I approached were polite and receptive, but one interaction at a Cervical Spine Research Society conference left a bad taste in my mouth. At lunchtime, I approached a table of six surgeons, all leaders in the field. I knew them from other conferences where I had seen them deliver lectures; they all held high academic positions. I politely asked if I could take five minutes of their time. No one said anything, so I started presenting my device.

One of the professors was from Dallas and had given a lecture at another conference about the difficulties of long scoliosis surgeries in the elderly that had greatly inspired me. I was especially eager to get his input; I respected his medical acumen. One minute into my presentation, one of the surgeons, who was from Denver, stopped and ferociously attacked me. He accused me of being rude and intrusive. The surgeon from Dallas joined in with a rude remark. None of these professors had any interest in hearing about my device. I stopped, apologized, and left the table, feeling quite dejected. So much for intellectual curiosity. Even to this day, it shocks me at how closed-minded my orthopedic surgeon colleagues can be.

Fortunately, not all surgeons are hostile to new ideas. I presented my device to the Congress of Neurological Surgeons in 2015 and I am proud to say that it won the Innovations Showcase, which means that the surgeons in charge determined that my device was worthy enough to be presented to the neurosurgical community.

This was a lifetime achievement for me that went without any celebration. I don't think you will ever come across any other surgeon who has had this accomplishment. Other competitors in the innovation showcase were multi-billion-dollar companies with endless resources. I had a working prototype, and my team had achieved a remarkable milestone. We had created a device from the ground up that was stronger than anything we have ever had—and much simpler.

I almost felt amused when I kept seeing surgeons' reactions to my comment. I would present my device at innovation showcases and tell them that my device was stronger than pedicle screws, and they would react as if I was talking crazy. I would tell them, look, you can make the screw so strong that it can hold this building. But if you put it in a junky, weak, and spongy bone, then what you get is junk. My device may not be as strong as a screw, but it holds on to very strong bone in a way that a screw cannot.

How did this research and invention uncover a seemingly major conspiracy in spine surgery? As I was inventing my device and developing it, I was learning more and more about biomechanics of the spine. The issues that I was facing also existed in pedicle screws, except no one talked about it. I was able to solve those issues in my device. Yet they remain unsolved in pedicle screw systems.

When I did my literature search, I was stunned to find out that the great majority of research says that screws did not work. Only Dr. Zdeblick's paper indicated that the screws worked great. As I dug deeper, the plot thickened. At the time, I felt as if I was living in a movie. How could all these facts be explained? This was the biggest question in my mind for the three years.

Sometimes people ask me how much work I put into creating my system, and I have a hard time putting a precise number on that. My wife is an attorney, and she can answer such questions precisely and easily. She litigates nursing home abuse cases, and the number of hours worked is a very easily calculated parameter. However, when you try to answer the same question regarding inventing a device, you cannot put a fixed number of hours on it. It was in my mind 24–7. Sometimes I dreamed about something, and when I woke up, I magically had the answer.

Of course, my wife must deal with the fact that my mind is constantly working on problems even when I'm not in the office. My life consists of being at work and being at home, but I have a hard time leaving my mind at the office. My only hobby is flying, which I do with my family, but my physical body exists in one place while my mind is in another. I readily admit that I am obsessed with solving medical problems. I cannot turn my brain off; it is on all the time.

To answer these questions, I had to innovate first. When I dug deep into spine surgery literature to learn more about biomechanics, I realized there was a significant void. All I could find was literature regarding the biomechanics of screws that had nothing to do with the behavior of the spine under stress. For three years, I had to innovate, research, and write the biomechanics that were specific to the spine. This was the only way I could get the answers I was looking for. So many times I found myself awake at 4:00 a.m.,pacing around our living room.

Only after researching, writing, and studying all the available spine literature, and turning the issues over in my mind for three years, did the issues come into focus. I finally realized the big mistake we as spine surgeons had made. Treating the spine as a subspecialty of orthopedics caused us to go down the wrong road and make poor choices. My conclusion after an exhaustive literature search and years of experimentation is that spine surgery was never meant to be a subspecialty of orthopedics or neurosurgery because spine surgery has its own complex biomechanics. After all, the spine is a complex mechanical device. This critical determination has broad implications, which I will describe in the following chapter.

CHAPTER SEVEN

~

How Spine Surgery
Went Off Track

As much as it pains me to admit this, spine surgeons—myself included—failed our patients. It is incredibly distressing. I became a doctor and went into medicine because I sincerely want to help people. I didn't realize until many years into my career that my clinical training suffered from a systemic flaw. Because of that defect, I had learned procedures and methods from well-meaning instructors who passed on erroneous information to generations of spine surgeons. None of us students thought too deeply about the underlying reasons for doing what we did. Why would we? If smart, talented, dedicated, and honest individuals wrote medical textbooks based on rigorous scientific study, who were we neophytes to question them? I was at the very top of my class in medical school, ranked number one in my first two academic years, which meant that I studied and learned my textbooks *better* than my peers. The words might just as well have been written on slabs of stone; such was my faith in the spine surgery leadership.

What's interesting is how we got to this place. As medicine evolved over many decades, spine surgery became a subspecialty of neurosurgical or orthopedic surgery, which became composed of two separate subspecialties itself. It is crucial to understand the difference between the two subspecialties of spine surgery. I believe the failure of the leaders of the field to understand this important topic is one of the factors that has derailed the practice.

One subspecialty is called "deformity surgery," which is actually how spine surgery started. Initially the diagnostic tool we had was X-rays, with which we could see bones and the curvature of the spine. The first surgeries performed on the spine in the 19th century—even before scoliosis surgeries—were done to correct deformity in patients suffering from tuberculosis.

In this subspecialty of the spine, X-rays now make the diagnosis easy. We know what the normal curvature of the spine is. Using the frontal view, when you look from the front to the back of the spine, it should be straight. When you look at the spine from the side, there are three curvatures: one in the cervical spine, one in the thoracic spine, and one in the lumbar spine.

There are different theories as to why the upright human being has developed these curvatures. I hypothesize that the cervical and lumbar lordosis and thoracic kyphosis is present to house organs such as the lungs, heart, and abdominal contents. It would be very inefficient for load-carrying if the organs grew on both sides of the spine. To house the lungs, the thoracic spine needs to fall into kyphosis. To compensate for that, the cervical and lumbar spine fall into lordosis to provide balance and make the paraspinal muscles work most efficiently.

Based on measurements over decades, we know what degree the curvatures should be in the general public. However, in a condition called scoliosis, the spine comes out of balance. This could occur under different types of conditions, but, in scoliosis, the spine twists on itself. Therefore, the deformity is in three dimensions.

We know what normal is for the curvature of the spine, and we know what abnormal is, and diagnosis of deformity is made with X-rays. The surgery is highly technical and requires a very long fusion spanning regions of the spine. Such a surgery might take ten to twelve hours and may require a team of surgeons, possibly even staged surgery.

I call the next subspecialty of spine surgery "true spine surgery" because it comprises 90 percent of the surgeries performed and is always done to treat pain. A typical patient in this category is a forty-five-year-old mechanic who lifts a heavy weight and sustains an injury to an intervertebral disc, causing it to herniate and pinch the nerve, leading to severe back and leg pain. As I've mentioned, we did not have a true understanding of what happens to the intervertebral discs until the invention of the MRI. With that tool, we were finally able to look at the soft tissue, especially in the intervertebral discs, and see the extent of the damage. Before the MRI, it was extremely difficult to assess the discs, and we had to inject dye around the nerves to see if they were being pinched. It can be argued that the invention of the MRI marked the beginning of spine surgery.

Compared to deformity surgery, true spine surgery is less difficult because when damage occurs to the spine, it happens in a localized area. There is no rule that says that only one area can get damaged in an accident or from trauma, but it is usually one area that causes most of the pain. Therefore, the surgery required to relieve the pain is in a localized area and far smaller than scoliosis surgery.

There is a very important aspect of this subspecialty of the spine that many people fail to appreciate: the diagnosis. A correct diagnosis in spine surgery to treat pain is extremely difficult. Sometimes when you look at an MRI, all the discs are intact and healthy except one. In that situation, it is relatively easy to find the source of the pain. But very frequently, an MRI will show two or three discs that are damaged. In that situation, it is hard to determine which disc is the source of the pain or which disc contributes to overall pain and to what extent.

As I have explained in previous chapters, we know that pain in the spine is generated by inflammation. However, we do not have a diagnostic study to see the relative amount of inflammation or the location of the inflammation. In this subspecialty of spine surgery, the surgery itself is not difficult relative to scoliosis surgery, but the diagnosis can be extremely difficult. That is one of the reasons that spine surgery sometimes gets a bad reputation. As surgeons, we tend to operate on the worst-looking disc. However, it is a well-known fact in the world of spine surgery that when you have two discs next to each other, or possibly separated by some healthy discs, the one that looks the worst is often *not* the source of the pain, and the one that does not look as bad might be affecting the patient. With the diagnostic tests we currently have available, the correct diagnosis remains elusive.

As a spine surgeon who has been in practice for twenty years, I learn something from every patient I treat. Correctly diagnosing the source of pain is almost an art form acquired over a long career. Every complaint I hear from a patient is a clue, and every little problem the patient describes is a hint. This includes the way the patient walks and stands. These clues add up to come up with the best diagnosis.

Very busy spine surgeons—often those who are technically the best—use physician assistants or others to help manage their patients. This means that many patients are not evaluated by the surgeon but by a physician assistant. I do not want to complain about my colleagues using physician assistants in their practice, as sometimes there is no other choice. I think about hiring PAs every time I'm in the clinic. I know, of course, if money were a priority, that I could significantly boost my income by using physician assistants. However, once you start doing that, and once you start decreasing contact with patients, I believe you stop learning and increase the risk of missing telltale signs and symptoms.

Spine surgery is not like other specialties. With some other conditions, such as diabetes, high blood pressure, or eye conditions, patients have relatively similar presentations. After a few years of practice, the physician's job becomes more or less routine and repetitive. In the world of spine surgery, every patient is different. There is no bell curve distribution of patients along the disease process. The distribution is more like a flatline throughout the population, which means that everybody is different. There is no normal that we can compare everybody to.

To make things even more complex, everyone's expectations are very different. Some patients expect a surgical procedure to eliminate pain and return their skeletal health to that of a twenty-year-old's. Those individuals are sometimes disappointed. Other patients who have been in pain for years or decades don't believe that any procedure will bring relief. More often than not, such individuals are pleasantly surprised, but only if they find a surgeon who takes the time to accurately diagnose and treat the source of their problem.

The majority of surgeons who perform deformity surgery practice in an academic setting. These surgeons publish papers, write textbooks, and give lectures, and we call them the leaders of the field. Most of their practice is scoliosis, which accounts for only ten percent of the spine surgeries being performed. These leaders of the field are practicing based on their experience with their patients, and that means scoliosis has a much larger influence on their decision-making and understanding of the spine. In turn, scoliosis affects the outcome, understanding, and teaching of the entire world of spine surgery in a disproportionate way. This is important to understand because it plays a key role in the reason that spine surgery is stuck in a dead end.

A Brief History of Spine Surgery— Or How We Got Here

One of the earliest spine surgeries was performed in the early 1900s. At that time, tuberculosis was a rampant and common disease that significantly deformed the spine. The first attempts to correct the problem were made by a surgeon in New York who fused the spine and stopped it from progressing into deformity. The results were not very good, and there were significant concerns about the surgeries. One of the biggest problems, besides lack of proper anesthesia, was that there was no good way of immobilizing the spine for the fusion to take place. Up until the 1950s, external bracing was used to keep the deformity aligned until the fusion could solidify the spine in the corrected position. Unfortunately, the external immobilization was very inefficient and often failed.

In the 1950s and 1960s, Dr. Paul Harrington came out with the first true instrumentation of the spine, called the Harrington rod. This was a ratcheted device with a hook on each end. Dr. Harrington placed the instrument on the side of the spine that was bending (concave side) and actually spread apart the spine to make it straight. This was a very important step in the treatment of scoliosis. In the 1970s and 1980s, Dr. Eduardo Luque from Mexico came up with wires that went under the lamina and were twisted over a straight rod. That brought the spine to the straight rod and resulted in a better correction than the Harrington rod by itself. By the 1970s and 1980s, there were hooks that hooked on to the lamina to distract and compress for a better correction. Then, in the mid-1980s, two surgeons in France placed a large screw into the vertebrae to be used as an anchor. That was the beginning of the pedicle screw system. In the mid-to-late 1980s, at the American Academy of Orthopaedic Surgeons, the surgeons from France presented their screw concept. From the late 1980s on, the pedicle screw gained significant traction in the treatment of scoliosis and continues to this day to be the most accepted way of treating this condition.

The reason that pedicle screws became so popular in the treatment of scoliosis was simply that they were superior to sublaminar wires and hooks. And most importantly, their use was in line with what we practice in general orthopedics and trauma. The pedicle screw was the first device that anchored directly to the spine, so it had a much better grip on the vertebral body. Scoliosis is a three-dimensional deformity, and the pedicle screw was able to correct the curvature of the scoliotic spine and also able to de-rotate some of the vertebrae. That provided a better three-dimensional correction.

For obvious reasons, the pedicle screw became the standard of care for treatment of scoliosis; it simply worked better in correcting scoliotic curve than the alternatives. X-rays of patients before and after surgery are impressive, and patients and surgeons take great satisfaction in seeing dramatic results.

Here's where the problem starts. In the world of spine surgery, it is very obvious that a significant problem has been solved with the use of pedicle screws to correct scoliosis, but also new problems arise. The new problems occur at both the bottom and the top of the rods. At the bottom, we constantly have to go to the pelvis for stronger fixation. At the top of the rods, we have a problem called *proximal junctional kyphosis*. This could mean a nonunion, and this is well known to surgeons. Pedicle screws, in conjunction with rods, may have worked better than hooks or wires or a combination of both, but they came with their own set of issues.

In the mid-1980s and early 1990s, the pedicle screw came into use not only for scoliosis correction but also for fusion surgeries. Up until that point, we had a significant problem with nonunion, so spine surgeons who had success with screws in scoliosis patients tried them on others. There were many patients in which the fusion would not heal, and they required a second or maybe even a third surgery. And so orthopedic spine surgeons started using screws as an adjunct for fusion surgeries.

Initially the results were not good, and there was significant skepticism about the use of these pedicle screws in disc fusion surgery. Still, it is apparent that in the early 1990s, there was a significant argument in academic circles about the use of pedicle screws as an adjunct in fusion surgeries. Also, there were many lawsuits due to the poor outcomes—about 7,000 of them. As a result, the FDA did not approve these pedicle screws to be used for fusion surgeries.

Then in 1993, as I mentioned in Chapter Five, a spine surgeon from the University of Wisconsin published a preliminary paper that was authored by him alone, stating that pedicle screws worked beautifully.

When I went looking for the final report, I was told by a medical professor that the surgeon in question abandoned the study and did not finish it. I cannot prove that, but it appears to be the case. Over the next several years, there were six prospective, randomized studies by other authors that said these screws do not work as an adjunct to fusion surgeries, but surgeons ignored those results.

After Zdeblick's preliminary study was published, lawsuits regarding pedicle screws disappeared, and their use became more accepted based on that paper. This is where the story gets interesting. Why did the lawsuits end? Why did doctors believe a preliminary report and ignore six later studies that disproved pedicle screw efficacy?

As mentioned, many of the leaders in the field who are surgeons have academic positions, publish papers, and give lectures at meetings. And, importantly, they are scoliosis surgeons; therefore, they are greatly influenced in their work by the success they have achieved using pedicle screws to correct scoliosis. The scoliosis field of spine surgery, despite being only about one in ten spine surgeries, has a disproportionate impact on the overall field of spine surgery, almost to the point that scoliosis surgery has ruined the rest of spine surgery.

Scoliosis surgeons have been fooled into believing that the pedicle screw is a great anchor. However, even in scoliosis, there are problems with it. I have talked to many scoliosis surgeons and raised the issues of pedicle screws. They say that they could not do surgery without the pedicle screws and that they work great for scoliosis surgery. They are unwilling to believe that the screws that work so well in scoliosis are anything but the best option for all other spine surgeries.

Smart people can and do still make dumb mistakes. Pedicle screws work great in scoliosis because the curvature is in the middle of the construct. The pedicle screw works to distribute the force along many screws, and all the screws share the burden to correct the deformity. The problem with pedicle screws is at the top and the bottom of the construct, where they show their true weakness. This problem is not unique to the rest of spine surgery. There are also significant problems in scoliosis because of the same issue.

As the patient's age goes up into the forties and fifties, scoliosis surgery has to extend beyond the spine into the pelvis for better purchase and, at the top, it has to go up all the way to T4. The problem with pedicle screws in general spine surgery is also present in scoliosis. However, the scoliosis surgeons are fooled by the power of the pedicle screw in correcting the curvature and leading to satisfactory X-rays. They cannot see the shortcomings of the screws at the top and the bottom of the construct.

As I mentioned above, one of the major problems in scoliosis surgery is proximal junctional kyphosis. Not to get into too much detail, but proximal junctional kyphosis is a direct side effect of using pedicle screws to correct scoliosis. Surgeons did not believe their eyes. They continued to believe that the screws were magic and worked well, even when they did not.

After his paper was published, Dr. Zdeblick received, according to a US Senate investigation, $34 million over the next fifteen years from an instrument company, Medtronic, that was at the center of lawsuits.

Dr. Zdeblick was in charge of another very important study around 2005. This was the study of a product called *bone morphogenic protein* (BMP), which is a bone substitute sold by the same instrument company, Medtronic, as a substitute for a bone graft.

BMP is a hormone that we all have. When we break a bone, it is excreted in the fracture site, and it promotes healing of the bone. This protein was identified in the 1960s, and it was later manufactured in a laboratory. The Medtronic product, named Infuse, avoids the need for bone grafting and bone harvesting, which is a big deal in spine surgery. Dr. Zdeblick was the main author in evaluating the BMP. I believe there were significant problems with his reporting of the side effects of the product. (Dr. Zdeblick denied that his research failed to disclose important information.)

Between 2002, when BMP-2 was approved by the FDA, and 2014, more than 1 million people worldwide received the biologic drug.

During that time, several medical journals published results of studies that presented favorable data. Not all spine surgeons were convinced, however, that Infuse was completely safe. In June 2011, *The Spine Journal* devoted most of its issue to a review of the use of BMP-2. An editorial co-authored by Dr. Carragee of Stanford University School of Medicine noted that there were many issues surrounding BMP-2 that had been glossed over: "After the original industry-sponsored trials for recombinant human bone morphogenetic protein-2 (rhBMP-2), which were remarkable for the complete absence of reported rhBMP-2-related clinical adverse events, there came many reports of complications by authors unsponsored by the promoting company."

That *The Spine Journal* issue also caught the attention of major news organizations. According to a 2011 article in the *Wall Street Journal*:

The medical journal that published two of the four papers on which Dr. Burkus was lead author, the *Journal of Spinal Disorders & Techniques*, was edited by Thomas Zdeblick, an orthopedic surgeon at the University of Wisconsin School of Medicine and Public Health who has received more than $24 million from Medtronic since 2001. Dr. Zdeblick was a co-author on both papers, but disclosed no financial relationship with Medtronic in the papers. He didn't respond to calls seeking comment. In a forthcoming letter to the editor he recently sent to *Spine*, Dr. Zdeblick said that none of the payments he received from Medtronic were directly related to Infuse® but that he receives royalties for a cage that Infuse is placed in when it's inserted in the spine. Dr. Kuntz [Medtronic chief medical & scientific officer and senior VP] says Medtronic now prohibits researchers who receive royalties from it to conduct clinical trials aimed at obtaining FDA approval for Medtronic products." [Medtronic has denied any wrongdoing in connection with its relationship with Dr. Zdeblick.]

More inquiries into potential adverse effects of BMP-2 followed, which ultimately led to the filing of a large number of lawsuits nationwide, as well as scrutiny of the doctors who wrote favorable articles and who also received payments or compensation from the manufacturer. A portion of the sums Dr. Zdeblick received from Medtronic formed the basis of allegations in an Infuse bone graft lawsuit filed against Medtronic in 2013, one of many filed against the company for allegedly promoting the product for uses for which it did not have FDA approval. The plaintiff sued Medtronic because he "suffered grievous personal injuries as a direct and proximate result of Defendants' (Medtronic's) misconduct." Background information in this case about payments Medtronic made to several orthopedic surgeons came from a Senate investigation in 2008. Dr. Zdeblick was not a party to the lawsuit against Medtronic; he was named as one of many "opinion leaders" who received payments from Medtronic, his being the largest amount noted. The following are allegations made in the lawsuit, which was settled without a finding of wrongdoing against either Medtronic or Dr. Zdeblick:

> Thomas A. Zdeblick, M.D., the Chairman of the Department of Orthopedics and Rehabilitation at the University of Wisconsin, received over $19 million from MEDTRONIC from 2003 to 2007 for consulting services and royalty payments. Although Dr. Zdeblick only disclosed annual payments exceeding $20,000 in University conflict of interest forms, he actually received between $2.6 and $4.6 million per year. In 2007 alone, Dr. Zdeblick received $2,641,000 in consulting fees from MEDTRONIC. From 1998 through 2004, Dr. Zdeblick was paid an annual salary of $400,000 by MEDTRONIC under a contract that only required him to work eight days per year at a MEDTRONIC site in Memphis, Tennessee, and to participate in "workshops" for surgeons.

Dr. Zdeblick also has been a significant contributor to MEDTRONIC's promotion of Infuse®, authoring seven peer-reviewed articles on rhBMP-2 and appearing as a presenter at medical conferences and symposia in which the topics included discussion of off-label uses of the product. On a MEDTRONIC-owned website, "www.Back.com," Dr. Zdeblick describes the advantages of Infuse® and appears in an online video discussing the benefits of the product.

In 2013, as detailed in a *New York Times* article, an outside review of Medtronic's clinical data found that its spinal treatment's benefit was overstated. The article notes that Dr. Zdeblick defended his work and insisted his ties to Medtronic had not influenced him. Further, Dr. Zdeblick said in a statement that he had not misrepresented any findings.

In 2014, Medtronic paid $22 million to settle approximately 1,000 legal claims arising over Infuse and set aside $140 million for future expected claims. In making the settlement, Medtronic made the following statement: "This agreement is a compromise of disputed claims and is not in any way an admission of liability or validity of any defense in the litigation of Medtronic. The company continues to stand behind Infuse® Bone Graft…and will vigorously defend the product and company actions in the remaining cases."

It is important for me to note that, to the best of my knowledge, neither Dr. Zdeblick nor Medtronic were ever found guilty of any wrongdoing in these matters by any court, and both Dr. Zdeblick and Medtronic have strenuously denied wrongdoing in connection with all of the research studies and business arrangements discussed herein. The US Senate completed a thorough investigation but again, to the best of my knowledge, never sanctioned or reprimanded Medtronic nor any of the spine surgeons who received the company's payments. Those who are interested in learning more about the controversy will find ample reading material online. I have opinions about the controversy based on my own medical and scientific experience and training, and I have many unanswered questions.

Academic doctors must have high ethics, and I believe there are significant issues with Dr. Zdeblick's research. (As noted, Dr. Zdeblick stands behind the validity of his research.) Once there are issues regarding ethics in one study, it should automatically bring the previous work into question. I believe that all my colleagues would agree that the paper Dr. Zdeblick published in 1993 completely changed the course of spine surgery. Many questions need to be answered before we move forward. Why was this paper published as a preliminary report? Why was it never finished? Did this coincide with the lawsuits for the instrument companies? Did the disappearance of the lawsuits coincide with the millions that Dr. Zdeblick reportedly received from Medtronic? The most important issue is that Dr. Zdeblick's work has so far never been duplicated, even after six independent, multicenter, multiauthor, research articles.

To make matters worse, there was another article, a much-anticipated paper, published in *Spine* in December 2018. The authors looked at the outcome of spinal fusions with and without screws, and they found that the addition of screws did not improve outcomes whatsoever. (*Spine*, 2018 December 1; 43(23); 1619-30). To this day, with this seventh article stating that pedicle screws do not work, I am baffled that the entire world of spine surgery ignores a mountain of evidence. The big question is, why?

Instrument companies have a death grip on the world of spine surgery. The great majority of leaders of the field in academic positions are also consultants for these instrument companies. When you become a consultant, I believe this means you are not a scientist anymore. It seems to me that you are now an undercover operative who is trying to advance the agenda of the big instrument companies. It has come to the point that no number of research papers or any amount of evidence will convince these consultants that there is a significant problem with the instrumentation and techniques used in the world of spine surgery today. The research continues to accumulate, but we just keep trucking along as if nothing has happened.

A Dead End

While I can and do blame the instrument companies for keeping us here at a dead end, it is orthopedic spine surgeons themselves who are responsible for getting us here. In the 1950s, 1960s, and 1970s, all surgical specialties improved. The biggest part of it had to do with improved anesthesia techniques, which allowed surgeons to safely perform lengthy surgeries.

In the 1950s and 1960s, a German-Swiss team developed principles for long bone fracture fixation in orthopedic surgery, called AO principles (AO stands for Arbeitsgemeinschaft für Osteosynthesefragen). These principles advocate rigid fixation of the fracture ends to promote healing together, and this idea spread throughout the world. By the 1980s, we were fixing fractures in the extremities using hardware by placing plates and screws spanning the fracture site to hold the ends together rigidly, and these worked very well. This technique reduced the healing time without the need for lengthy cast immobilization, and return to function was very good.

Around the same time, in the 1970s and 1980s, fusion surgery was becoming very common in spine surgery, which is a subspecialty of orthopedic surgery. When pedicle screws appeared in the mid-1980s, they were very consistent with the principles of AO that we had already implemented in long bone fracture fixation with great success. The same concept of rigid fixation was transferred from general orthopedics to the world of spine surgery. The biggest evidence for this statement is the presence of a major society in the world of spine surgery called "AO Spine," which is basically promoting rigid fixation using screws and rods. This short history lesson is important because it shows how young the field of spine surgery is. You might believe that operations to relieve back pain using rods and screws were done a hundred years ago, but that's not the case. The entire subspecialty of back surgery to address pain started within the past forty years.

In the early 1990s, when surgeons applied pedicle screws to spinal fusion, the results were not as clear cut as fracture fixation. There were initially quite a number of suboptimal and sometimes flat-out bad results. As noted earlier, there were lawsuits for using these pedicle screws, and the FDA initially refused to approve them for use in the spine as an adjunct to fusion surgery. At the peak of disagreement about the use of pedicle screws, Dr. Zdeblick published his paper.

Spine surgery was very young, and decisions about what direction to go were being made. In my opinion, Dr. Zdeblick's paper caused the entire world of spine surgery to follow the principles of general orthopedic long bone fracture fixation principles and go in the direction of rigid fixation using hardware, including pedicle screws and rods. By the time the six other papers came out saying that the pedicle screws are ineffective in increasing fusion rates and definitely ineffective in changing the outcome of the surgery, instrument companies had a firm grip on the entire world of spine surgery.

Instrument companies currently dictate everything we do in spine surgery. It is a fact that companies are constantly importing technology from general orthopedics to spine surgery. This has caused a series of failed technologies and inventions that come and go with no clear advantage to the patient. Not everyone loses, of course. The implantation of devices enriches instrument companies and their CEOs to the tune of tens of billions of dollars each year.

Time to Own Our Mistakes

It is time to own our mistakes and correct what we, as spine surgeons, have done to our patients in performing complex spinal surgeries. The spine is a very different entity from a long bone fracture. The deforming forces are different, the makeup is different, and of course, the biology is very different. The principles that worked in fracture fixation will not work in the spine because the physics, mechanics, and anatomy are all different.

An extremely important factor that is often overlooked by academics is basic anatomy. The vertebra is a very complex bone, and it is not that simple to immobilize a very complex bone. With the AO technique, we have chosen the worst way.

You will recall that the vertebral body is composed of two types of bone: the cortical bone, which is the outside shell, and the cancellous bone, which is the inside spongy bone. Pedicles screws use the spongy, weak bone as an anchor. Right away, we are using a suboptimal area to grip the vertebra to immobilize it.

The most important flaw in the field of spine surgery is not understanding and not using biomechanics specific to the spine.

I attend spine conferences twice a year. I did my training at Harvard University under world-renowned surgeons. Not once at any spine conference I attended was there any discussion about biomechanics specific to the spine. Each time there was a lecture on biomechanics, the topic was based on the properties of the screw. These included the core, the length, the diameter, and the pitch of the screws. Those are topics unrelated to the spine. The experts were singularly focused on the biomechanics of the screw and not the biomechanics of the spine. I have yet to attend a single lecture or hear a surgeon talk about the true forces that we are trying to neutralize in the spine.

If you ask a spine surgeon how screws fail, there is a standard answer that it is a combination of toggle (side-to-side stress) and pullout. It is true that the only two options are toggle and pullout, but which one is the primary cause? The answer to this question is very important, because if you try to augment and make a device resistant to a secondary event, the primary event is going to go untreated, and the device is going to fail regardless of what you are trying to do. In any system, if there is a primary or secondary mode of failure, all of the efforts should be to counter and resist the primary event.

In my opinion, we should focus on the motion of the vertebra. In the next chapter, I will be going over the biomechanics of the spine in detail. However, I would like to say here that the motion of the vertebra is based on a rotational motion, with the axis through the middle of the disc space relative to the vertebra below. This means that the motion the pedicle screws have to stop is a rotational motion. One vertebra, relative to the vertebra below, does not slide back and forth, nor does it slide up and down. It rotates through the axis that runs through the middle of the disc space. Therefore, it is very simple to see that toggle is the primary mode that causes these screws to come loose as opposed to pullout. As shown in Figures 28 and 29 below, even surgeons can be fooled into thinking that a screw has pulled out. However, in this case the motion is purely rotational, and toggle is the primary failure mode.

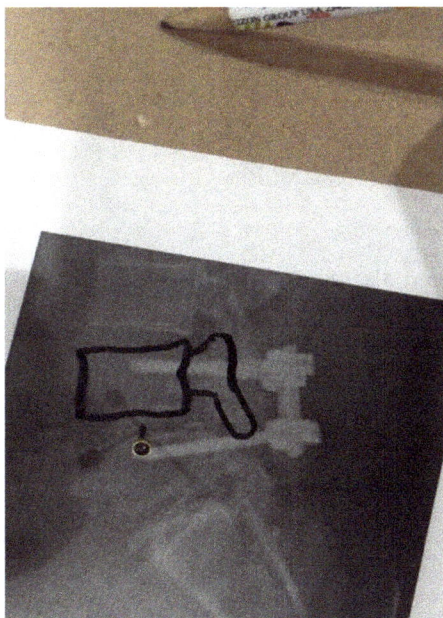

Figure 28: I Have Outlined the Vertebrae Above

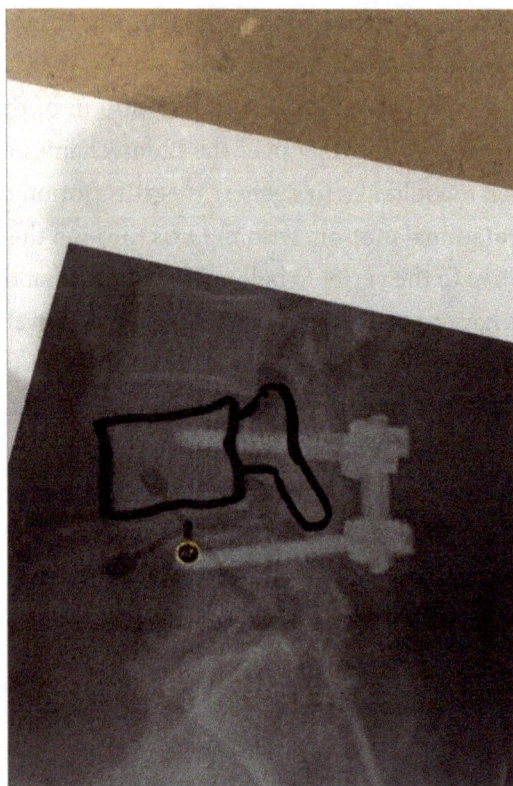

**Figure 29: I Have Rotated the Overlay Around the
Axis in the Middle of the Disc Space**

I have reviewed almost the entirety of the spine literature; I have read lectures and attended lectures about biomechanics. Everything we have done in the world of spine surgery within the last three decades has been to increase and improve the pullout strength of the screw. This has been achieved in multiple ways. Some screws are expandable. Some screws are fenestrated so that glue is shot through the core of the screw to come out from the holes along the screw. Once the cement squeezes out of the side holes, it turns into spikes that hopefully will hold on to the vertebra better. A review of the literature shows that everything we have done to improve and measure the function of the pedicle screw is the pullout strength. Each time there is talk about the pedicle screw construct in the spine, we talk about the pullout strength and the insertional torque. However, those topics are entirely irrelevant if the screws fail as a result of toggle.

Let's take more time to discuss "insertional torque." This is one of the most important measurements taken in spine literature to assess the strength of the pedicle screw construct. Insertional torque is proportional to the screw-bone interface. The more the screw gets inserted into the bone, the more the insertional torque goes up in a linear fashion. As the surgeon inserts the screw into the vertebra, they feel an increase in insertional torque, and basically the grip gets better and better. This gives the surgeon a false sense of security that the patient is obtaining a solid construct with the screw.

In actuality, the most important feature of using pedicle screws is that a screw inside the body has to stop toggle. When the rotational force is applied to the screw, this force does not get distributed evenly along the length of the screw. There are pressure points along its the length. This makes the failure of the bone-screw construct much more likely. The pedicle screw fools the surgeon who is inserting it, giving them the perception of great fixation. However, the patient is not getting what the surgeon thinks the patient is getting.

I believe this is an extremely important point because it puts a wedge between the surgeon and the patient. The surgeon is under the impression that the construct is very strong and that he has done a great job, but the patient has not received a construct as strong as the surgeon believes. When the patient comes back and there is a nonunion, the surgeon tends to blame the patient for the failure. But it is the construct that is weak.

I have made the suggestion to my colleagues that the pedicle screw is the worst thing that ever happened to the spine surgeon. When they hear that, they are in shock that I have even mentioned it. As I have explained, nothing is worse than a surgeon being deceived into believing they are doing a good job. When the construct fails and the patient ends up with a nonunion, the surgeon cannot understand what has happened because his level of suspicion is not high enough.

The failure to apply and understand the true biomechanics of the spine has given surgeons a false perception that screws provide adequate fixation. In reality, they do not. To be honest, I cannot believe spine surgeons have gone this route. It baffles me. We use cancellous bone—spongy bone—which is weak bone, as an anchor point, and we expect the screw to stop toggle, which is it not made for. When the papers show that it does not work, we do not want to believe it. This is purely crazy. At this point, I am not sure how many more papers have to come out for spine surgeons to realize there is something wrong going on. I believe AO spine should be renamed.

A Dental Analogy

When I did a review of the medical literature, I asked myself if there is any other subspecialty that has been exposed to a similar situation. You would think that would be a long shot, but I found a comparison: the field of dentistry. I reviewed the literature for dentistry, and it turns out there is some information in that specialty relevant to spine surgery.

Placement of an implant in the jawbone has now become routine practice. However, when they were initially doing the implants, there was a high failure rate. A significant amount of research was done to find out the reason. Initially they suspected that it was the compression causing the implants to fail. However, after conducting research, it turns out it was not compression but toggle.

The conclusion was that the rim of the bone that surrounds the implant at the location of the insertion into the maxilla is the most sensitive area. This area is called "the crown." That bone can resist compression significantly, but it is extremely sensitive to toggle forces. That caused a significant change in the practice of dentistry. Originally, the practice was to place the implant and the crown at one visit. Now it has become a staged procedure. First, the dentist places the implant and lets the bone grow into it so that the implant will be stronger. After three weeks, the crown is placed. That significantly reduces the rate of implant failure.

These findings are actually in line with spine surgery. We place these large screws into the vertebral body and expose them to significant toggle forces. I can now say that the world of dentistry has shown us that bone is very sensitive to toggle forces. That information is very consistent with the research in the world of spine surgery showing that the screws are ineffective. When you look at the big picture, everything starts to make sense.

Spine Surgery Is a Special Case

The environment of the spine and the forces that it is exposed to in the body make spine surgery a special case. As noted earlier, rigid fixation of fracture ends is the tried, tested, and successful concept in orthopedics—to an extent. There is a very important point that stands out with the spine as opposed to long bone fracture fixation. The concept of rigid fixation can be implemented to long bone fracture fixations for one very important reason: if you have a construct that is not super strong and the surgeon thinks that construct needs to be protected, then the surgeon can eliminate gravity. In terms of the upper extremity, of course, you can put the patient in a sling. In terms of the lower extremity, you can put the patient in a cast and on crutches. However, when it comes to the spine, you cannot eliminate gravitational forces. You cannot suspend the patient in the air. That means the construct you have placed in the spine is constantly exposed to many stresses.

Think of this situation as a high-rise building in an earthquake zone. You do not construct it to be stiff. We tried that, and it did not work. The tall building is made flexible. Very tall buildings can be placed on rollers so that when there is an earthquake, the building can flex and dissipate some of the forces.

The same concept should apply to the spine. As soon as we get up, we expose the spine to significant stresses. This could be true for a daily activity or a moderate amount of work. When the construct is a rigid fixation, there is a high chance of failure if there is a significant increase in stress momentarily.

The better way of doing the fixation is to have a device that can actually absorb high stresses and can flex and dissipate the stresses. I call this new technique and type of fixation *reactive-rigid fixation*. This is very important to understand. It is not rigid fixation and not flexible fixation but reactive-rigid fixation. The most optimal fixation device should not only hold the spine in a rigid fixation, but at times when there is increased stress, it should move and dissipate that stress. In that manner there will not be a catastrophic failure of the construct. This concept should be applied to fracture fixation as well. I think the world of orthopedic surgery needs to rethink their approach, too.

To have a reactive-rigid fixation, a material other than metal is required. Metal simply does not have the properties that can be both rigid and flexible. The alternative is to have a hybrid construct that is not only metal but also flexible material. I have had a difficult time discussing this with my orthopedic colleagues. For some reason, in orthopedic surgery, it has been hammered into our brains that the answer to any problem is a screw. Throughout general orthopedics, we have learned that we can place screws in any direction, at any distance, and at any angle with good results. That knowledge is applied to spine surgery, but it has had suboptimal results so far.

Training

Spine surgery is a subspecialty of neurosurgery and orthopedic surgery, which has implications for the ways in which new doctors are trained. When I was doing my orthopedic training, I spent very little time in spine rotations. When I was in spine rotation, I did not get to do anything or actually see anything during the surgery. I was standing there for hours on end and not really understanding what was going on in the surgery. After finishing my training, I did a fellowship in spine surgery but it was only one year. I cannot speak for all of neurosurgery, but I can see that exposure to biomechanics is likely minimal while studying brain surgery.

Sadly, in orthopedic surgery, we learned the wrong biomechanics, and this false information became imprinted in our brains. After I invented my device and won the Innovations Showcase in the Congress of Neurological Surgeons, I presented my device to different surgeons at conferences. My experience was very consistent throughout my endeavor: Neurosurgeons easily understood the principles and biomechanics of the spine as I explained it to them, and they were very receptive to the topic. Orthopedic spine surgeons were very different. I could not get them past the fact that a strap construct is in fact stronger than a screw-and-metal construct. Orthopedic spine surgeons are stuck believing that rigid fixation and screws are the ultimate devices for immobilization of the spine. This has been etched into their brains, and there is no changing it.

Each time I would tell a spine surgeon that my device that uses composite straps is stronger than the pedicle screw, they acted shocked and as if this were sacrilegious. However, my argument was very simple. You can make the screw strong enough to hold a building, but if it is placed in spongy bone, the construct is only as strong as the spongy bone can withstand. The device I invented uses composite flexible straps, which are stronger than the same size steel cable, but my device holds on to the very strong, very dense cortical bone as opposed to cancellous bone. Even though my device itself is not as strong as a screw, the actual construct is far stronger than the pedicle screw construct. I cannot make them understand that for some reason. It feels to me that if we are to move on from orthopedic surgery and perform spine surgery, surgeons will have to unlearn what they were taught and relearn the true biomechanics of the spine. The analogy would be like the difference between Newtonian and quantum physics. If someone is trying to study and use light properties and all they know is Newtonian physics, they would be lost. To truly study light and its properties, scientists need to learn quantum physics and build lasers.

With this statement, it almost sounds like I am backstabbing my colleagues. However, the truth needs to be told. Spine surgery is far too complex to be a subspecialty of orthopedic surgery or neurosurgery. In orthopedic surgery, you learn the wrong biomechanics and, in neurosurgery, I do not think you get exposed to enough biomechanics. If I have to pick between the two, I believe neurosurgeons have a much better chance of understanding the biomechanics of the spine because they have not been brainwashed with the rigid-fixation concept. Spine surgery should not be a subspecialty of any other surgery.

The big question, of course, is how it is possible that the world of spine surgery has gone in the wrong direction when a lot of patients are being treated by orthopedic spine surgeons and by neurosurgeons with very good results. How can that be explained? There are two levels to answer that question. First, the research says that patients are doing good, except the research also says we don't have to make the surgery super expensive to get the same results as a much cheaper surgery. To do so would be malpractice, because the standard of care is to use expensive equipment. The instrument companies sold not only the expensive equipment and devices to doctors and hospitals, but also the concept that their equipment is indispensable. But the truth is that none of the devices added any benefit to the patient. This is the concept that I've tried to discuss with my colleagues, but they are completely unwilling to consider that they have been duped.

The second issue is that the spine is a relatively stable structure to begin with, and that is why we have gotten away with it so far. The spine is a much more stable structure than we give it credit for. All of our learning in terms of surgical technique has come from fracture fixation. A fracture is a very unstable structure, but the spine by itself is a very stable structure. That's why, for so long, surgeons have gotten away with using incorrect biomechanics and instruments and still achieved good results.

Imperfection Is Progress; Instrument Companies Need to Come Clean

I have been going to neurosurgery and orthopedic spine surgery conferences twice a year since the start of my practice in 2002. In all those cases, I have never seen a surgeon get up and show a surgery in which he made a mistake or something bad happened in order to try to teach what went wrong. Not one time.

When I was in general surgery, we had a session called mortality-morbidity, which we called M&M. In those sessions, we presented mistakes we had made. Unfortunately, at the conferences I attend, the surgeons who are leaders in the field and in academic positions always show their best MRIs, best surgeries, and best outcomes. If they ever show a case that did not go very well, it seems to always be made to be some other surgeon's fault. That does not count. Showing a bad outcome or poor X-rays without knowing what happened during the surgery or the thought process does not help anyone. It is important for the surgeon who has made a mistake to present it and explain why he made that mistake and what happened that the case went wrong. This is sorely lacking in the world of spine surgery. When I go to those conferences, I get the picture that every procedure and every surgery goes very well and that there are absolutely no problems in spine surgery.

In the meantime, the research shows that we are not doing a good job. I once got up in front of six hundred surgeons at the American Academy of Orthopaedic Surgeons and said that we had created an alternative reality for ourselves. We have created a matrix in which everything is good. Meanwhile, outside of the matrix, our patients are not doing well. We have many patients who end up in pain management for the rest of their lives after having surgery.

In 2006, a new surgery called XLIF became available to us. XLIF stands for *extreme lateral interbody fusion*. This was a revolutionary surgery because doctors went in from the side instead of the front, and it was minimally invasive. I was actually the first surgeon in Northern California to perform this surgery. When the surgery became available, I had compiled experience with about 150 patients, and I was invited by an instrument company to give a lecture about the surgery to a room of spine surgeons. They asked me to present my experience with a few of these surgeries, so I picked nine surgeries that went perfectly. I also had another surgery that I contemplated presenting. In that surgery, I had placed the graft in a suboptimal position. It did not end up causing the patient any problems; however, the X-rays did not look good. I considered whether I should present that case or not, and I eventually decided that I should include my bad experience. In that particular instance, I recognized during surgery that the position was not optimal and tried to reposition the graft. However, it was stuck, and I broke the graft when trying to reposition it. My teaching point was that before insertion of the graft, it is important to have multiple X-rays and to make sure that the graft goes into the correct position.

I am very confident in my surgical technique, and I had no problem showing a room of spine surgeons my mistake. I presented my cases to a room of about fifty spine surgeons. The case in question was the tenth-last case I presented. When I put the X-rays on the podium, even I could not believe that it was my surgery. I explained exactly what happened. The patient had significant slippage of one vertebra over the other vertebra, and I kind of got lost. Even though the graft was well aligned with one of the vertebrae, it was not aligned with the other vertebra.

After my explanation, I was attacked by two spine surgeons who accused me of performing suboptimal surgery. But this was exactly why I was presenting this—so that they could learn from my mistake. If I only show the good cases, as everyone else does, I do not think it would teach as much as it would by my presenting of this case.

At the end of the lecture, I received applause that made me feel proud. It was more than the standard clapping that everyone receives at the end of a lecture. I was very happy with what I did, and I was comfortable in my own skin. I was happy that I had the courage to present my mistake and failure in front of fifty other spine surgeons. After my presentation, the company's CEO politely thanked me, but he did not even walk me out the door or downstairs. I got into my rental car and flew back to Sacramento, and I never heard from them again.

There are two culprits here. One is spine surgeons who are not presenting bad mistakes in conferences. One can almost not blame them, considering that peers can be unforgiving. The second culprit is the instrument companies who do not want something like that to happen. If there is a problem with a surgery, the immediate question is, which instrument was used? Every spine surgeon knows that poor outcomes, instrument failures, and patients who end up in pain management and on narcotics for the rest of their lives occur frequently. In the end, I blame the instrument companies for promoting such a culture among spine surgeons.

Most people are completely unaware of the role instrument companies play in controlling the entire world of spine surgery. I have been complaining about the misrepresentation of instruments in the world of spine surgery literature for a long time. When I arrived at my office one morning, I had the November 1, 2020, issue of *Spine* waiting for me. The lead article was very interesting and very disappointing. It was entitled, "Undisclosed Conflict of Interest Is Prevalent in Spine Literature."

If I have to define *bias* in this situation, it is the influence and the power of instrument companies taking spine surgeons in the direction that they want to. What I am about to say is a very well-known problem in spine surgery and not just my personal issue.

How do these companies achieve this power and influence? Of course, an instrument company cannot come up with the literature. They approach someone who is almost always a famous surgeon that holds an academic position, and who is often willing to bend to the company's demands. That surgeon becomes a "consultant" and basically gets on the instrument company's payroll. At that point, what should happen does not happen. Based on ethical and moral obligations, the surgeon should evaluate the products as they are. More often than not, they end up writing favorable articles to advance the interest of the company. Now, I do not want to accuse all academics involved with companies; I actually have a good number of academics who are on my side of the issue.

One good example is disc replacement. The fusion somehow comes as a very irreversible and destructive surgery to the spine. No one wants their spine to be fused and stiff. However, the surgery we had available was fusion, so the question was whether we have to fuse. In the 1980s, 1990s, and early 2000s, companies came out with disc replacement prostheses. There were very favorable early papers, but subsequent results were not good at all. Disc replacement did not perform well at all in the lumbar spine. Disc replacement is even very questionable in the cervical spine.

The influence instrument companies have over surgeons to produce favorable papers has to stop. As spine surgeons, we are doctors and scientists who have taken an oath to do everything we can for the benefit of our patients first. I cannot blame the instrument companies for the status of the world of spine surgery, but I do believe they are responsible for keeping us here and preventing true progress. This has been done through the use of so-called consultants.

As a surgeon, I am very close to my patients. I do not use any physician assistants or nurse practitioners in my practice. It has become difficult for me to inform my patients about the risks and benefits of surgery. Not only do we not know what to tell patients because we do not know who to believe, but we have probably been given false information for decades based on biased literature.

This is truly devastating to the field of spine surgery. I am not sure if exposing instrument companies will help patients to start trusting us again. But we have to move in that direction with our hearts in the right place, which is in the best interest of our patients. Correcting the behavior of so-called "consultants" is necessary to keep spine surgery at the highest level of ethics. Consultants need to realize that advancement of the instrument company agenda is not what they signed up for. They need to evaluate everything based on evidence, and they need to be impartial to the outcome of those studies.

In most medical specialties, medical companies have scientists working for them who innovate. For example, a drug company has chemists who come up with new medications. Then it is left to physicians to evaluate the new meds.

Spine surgery is a unique field. The spine is a mechanical device that operates based on certain principles. In this field, innovation should come from surgeons, because not only are we talking about a device, but also about the complex anatomy that surrounds it. You can have a good idea and make a device that works great in the lab, but if you try to put it inside a patient, it might not work. Therefore, the relationship between surgeon and instrument company should be protected.

Dream Big

Residency surgical training was an absolute nightmare. To this day, I wake up every so often in a sweat and shaking with a recurring nightmare that I have just been informed I have to repeat part of my residency. I understand that clinical professors have a duty to make us eliminate mistakes but, at some point, teaching turns into relentless abuse that permanently scars your brain. I have been in practice for twenty years now. I have done more than four thousand surgeries and have never been sued for any surgeries I have ever done. I always ask myself, was it necessary for my soul to burn and become permanently scarred for me to become a good surgeon?

As brutal as the experience was, one comment made to me by my chairman in my orthopedic residency had a profound beneficial effect on me. I was called into his office because one of my professors complained that I was constantly offering up new ideas instead of regurgitating the standard thinking in textbooks. After talking with me for about ten minutes, he finally said, "Ardavan, you are a dreamer. It is always the dreamers who come up with inventions; it's not those guys that win awards. If we didn't have dreamers, we would have nothing. I keep telling the junior professors, and they still don't get it." His advice to me was to keep dreaming big and ignore the narrow-minded.

I will never forget that comment. It became one of the driving forces for me when I started my research and development.

The root cause of the problem for spine surgery is the fact that there is no accountability from the instrument companies. The CEOs only have one objective, which is to make money for the company. A CEO can force a product onto the market without using the correct channels or the correct evaluation. The true nature of the product and its failures surfaces decades down the road. By then, the CEO has retired with a large amount of money. They cannot be held accountable at that point. However, there are millions of patients who have had procedures that are pretty much worthless. These patients have trusted their bodies to us as spine surgeons. Under no conditions, or for any amount of money, should a spine surgeon break that trust. The true progression in the field of spine surgery must occur with an impartial observation of data and interpretation of outcome without consideration of any monetary gain.

Now, by no means am I trying to say that we should evaluate a device thoroughly, then bring it to market. That can't happen. The best way is to expedite bringing products to market, but soon after have a thorough evaluation of the device.

This book will, I hope, bring awareness of the fact that the literature is biased, and we as spine surgeons have misunderstood the basic principles of spine surgery. Unfortunately, this has made spine surgery—in my opinion and in my interpretation of published research—into one of the biggest scams in the world of medicine. There is good news. I will present the solution in the next chapter and explain what needs to be done to put things back on the right track.

CHAPTER EIGHT

The Future of Spine Surgery

S pine surgery is at a dead end. If nothing is done to rectify the current situation, the medical specialty will remain there, much to the detriment of doctors and patients. The only beneficiaries of maintaining the status quo will be medical device companies that will continue to make billions of dollars selling unnecessary equipment to an unsuspecting public. With so much to lose, those companies will lobby hard to sway public opinion and convince you that everything is fine. They will tell you that a "crazy" doctor in Sacramento is tilting at windmills. You may safely ignore him.

Over the last four decades, there have been a significant number of inventions that have come and gone in the world of spine surgery. Every single one was auspicious when it came out. But after a decade of each being in use, it turned out that none of them made any impact in terms of improving the outcome for patients. As I explained in the previous chapter, we are currently using instruments that our research shows do not—improve patient outcomes. We have improved biologics as far as possible, but we still have not improved the overall outcome.

We have implemented to the spine what we learned from general orthopedic surgery. AO Spine is one of the biggest societies in spine surgery and the group that established general principles for fracture fix-ation starting in 1958. This includes the concept of rigid fixation using instruments. I have explained multiple times that this is something we should not have done. However, I agree with the implementation of this concept in the beginning because we had to start somewhere. At the time, we did not know what would and would not work in spine surgery until we tried it. I do not condemn the use of orthopedic surgery principles for spine surgery. But once we discovered a mountain of evi-dence that it did not work, we continued using it for reasons discussed in Chapter Seven.

What is most distressing is that, even if you look at fracture fixation principles, we did not employ those principles appropriately; we applied them blindly. For example, fracture fixation principles involve analysis of the fracture to see how stable it is. We always look at fracture displace-ment and try to counter the forces acting to displace the fracture. That is done by understanding muscle insertion into different parts of the bone and pulling the fracture fragments in different directions. Only by understanding those forces were we able to invent devices to counter those forces and achieve successful fixation leading to fracture healing.

That did not happen in the world of spine surgery. We never under-stood the forces that acted on the vertebra and how the vertebra is being affected by different forces and different directions. As noted, in twenty years of attending medical conferences, I have never heard anyone say that the goal of the instruments we are using today as an adjunct for fusion is to neutralize the forces on the vertebra. The vertebra is a very complex bone, and vital and dangerous structures surround it. The only thing we have done is to insert a device based on what the anatomy has allowed. This is without really understanding or studying the forces that are acting on the spine. I have said many times in this book that we have used can-cellous bone as an anchor, and we have expected the pedicle screw to stop toggle, which it cannot do. When papers are published showing evidence that the instruments do not work, we look the other way.

The spine's actual biomechanics can only be learned by studying the deforming forces that act on the vertebra. Understanding those forces will help people develop inventions, devices, and anchors with a chance of success.

Even if we understand the deforming forces and implement devices to counter those forces, how can the devices be applied and used safely without damaging the important structures around the vertebra? We not only have to consider biomechanics, but also consider the complex anatomy to determine if the anatomy allows for certain devices. Without understanding the biomechanics, the implementation of something just based on anatomy is also not the correct method.

Spine Biomechanics

The science of the forces that move the vertebral bone is called *biomechanics*. As I've discussed, the spine is comprised of three segments: cervical, thoracic, and lumbar. When you look from the front, the spine is straight. When you look from either side, we have three curvatures: cervical lordosis, thoracic kyphosis, and lumbar lordosis. I have also explained previously that these curves were most likely formed to accommodate the chest cavity, lungs, and heart.

The spine is a complex structure that moves in three-dimensional space. Motions of the spine include flexion, extension, lateral bending, and lateral rotation. Let's dissect each of these motions to see how they interrelate.

How often does someone find themselves bending sideways, or laterally? Not very often. It is a very uncomfortable position. How often does someone perform extension, or bend backward? It's a very unstable position, and we normally only engage in this for a short period of time. One example of performing extension would be changing a lightbulb on the ceiling. We spend the great majority of our time in flexion, or bending forward. From the time that we wake up to the time that we go to bed, just about everything we do is in flexion. When two fighters square off, they square off in partial flexion because that is the most stable position. When we engage in an activity such as working on an instrument or lifting an object, this is also done in flexion. Even when we are walking, the spine flexes forward. Therefore, we should focus on the flexion motion of the spine when studying the forces acting on the spine.

The major force that acts on the spine is gravity, which goes in one direction only. The other force that acts on the spine comes from the paraspinal muscles. The spine has very strong and very active extensor muscles, which are responsible for humans becoming upright mammals. The muscles that flex the spine are very weak, and they are much smaller, including the abdominal flexors. Most of the time, the spine flexes forward because of gravity.

The motion of the spine is extremely complex. When you deal with something complex, it should be broken down to the smallest unit that repeats itself. That allows for an understanding of the entire entity. The unit in the spine is composed of two vertebrae with a disc in between. We call this a *motion segment*. What happens in flexion of a motion segment? As the trunk moves forward, the whole center of gravity starts moving forward. This causes the spinal vertebrae to sequentially flex forward.

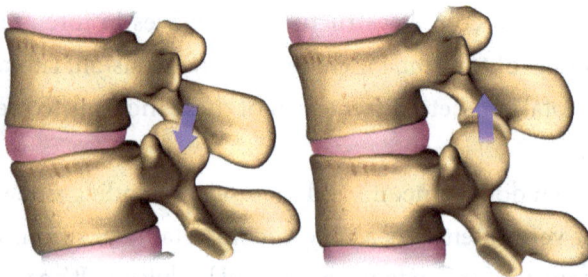

Figure 30: Vertebrae Flexion

It may sound simple now, but it took me five years to decode the motion of the spine. Let's assume we are talking about L4 over L5. L5 does not have any deforming capacity or force into the construct because it supports the construct. It is L4 that is flexing forward relative to L5. The deforming force that tends to flex the L4 forward comes from the vertebra above, which is L3. As L4 starts flexing forward, initially the disc collapses slightly in the front. Next, through the posterior longitudinal ligament, the vertebral body of L3 lifts the back of the vertebral body of L4. Therefore, L4 flexes forward. This motion is a rotational motion with the axis through the middle of the disc.

Let's now superimpose the medical device hardware over this motion. We can imagine that L4 and L5 are connected with pedicle screws into the vertebral body of L4 and the vertebral body of L5, and this is connected with one rod on each side. The screws are trying to stop the vertebral body of L4 from flexing forward. Now, here comes the problem. A screw is a device that is made to resist pullout. A screw works well when the force is distributed evenly along the length of the screw, and it can counter the forces that are parallel to its axis. That is not what is happening inside the human body. There, the motion that the screws are trying to stop is a rotational motion.

Such a situation is no different than a door that is jammed closed. If you want to open a stuck door, you do not try to push it close to the hinge; you try to push the edge farthest away from the hinge. This technique requires the least amount of force to move the jammed door. The same concept applies to vertebral motion. Imagine that you superimpose a record player over the motion segment between the two vertebrae, with the center of the record player over the center of disc rotation. I call this "Ardavan's record player." As you go away from the center of rotation, the forces decrease, and the motion increases. That means the most effective way to immobilize the moving record player is to hold on to the part that is farthest away from the center.

Once you superimpose a record player over our construct, including two vertebrae (L4 and L5 with the L4-5 disc between the hardware), you can draw a line from the center of the disc onto the different parts of the screw and calculate the amount of force each section of the screw is countering. This is very important because the force does not get distributed evenly along the length of the screw. The most effective area is the farthest away from the axis of rotation, which is the point of insertion of the screw into the vertebral body. If that bone fails at the point of insertion, as you come along the length of the screw, you get closer and closer to the axis of rotation, and that means the motion decreases and the force increases.

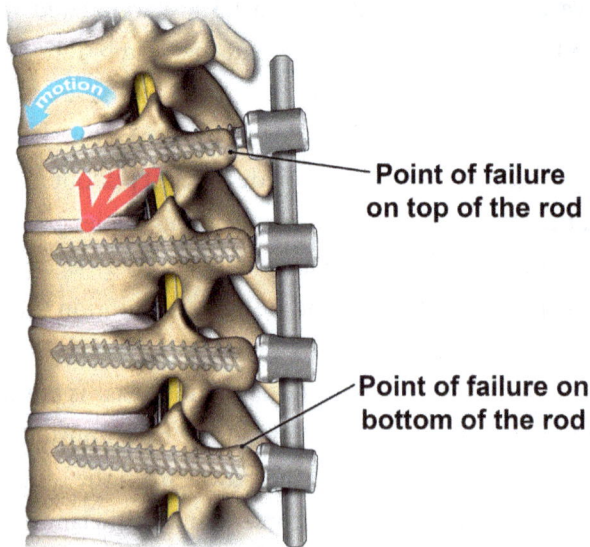

Point of failure on top of the rod

Point of failure on bottom of the rod

Figure 31: The rim of bone at the site of screw insertion is the primary fixation. That point is farthest away from the axis of rotation.

This is a very important concept to understand because the single point of maximum fixation is that rim of bone at the site of insertion. If that bone fails, the rest of the screw fails like a zipper, because as it goes closer to the axis, the force increases. This means the pedicle screw is not an effective way of immobilizing this motion. Not only that, but the screw has to do this using cancellous bone. As this cancellous bone passes through the pedicle into the vertebral body, it becomes nearly useless. Remember, the rim of bone at the site of insertion of the screw into the vertebral body is the primary fixation. That is it. If it fails, the entire screw will fail.

There is very strong evidence for this statement. Another technique for inserting screws into the vertebrae is with cortical screws. In this technique, a much smaller and shorter screw is used, but the trajectory is more medial to lateral. That is where the laminae get thicker. The technique has become more popular, and the reason for its success is that there is thicker cortical bone at the site of insertion. Of course, cortical screws create a new set of problems. I need to mention that this is the first time that someone has explained how these screws fail.

Generations of orthopedic surgeons, myself included, went about their business without giving the biomechanics of the spine much thought. We all probably believed that someone older, wiser, smarter, and more experienced had figured it all out, which is why they told us to do it this way. Again, I can't blame them. When something is written by great authorities in medical textbooks, it's hard to push back. We presume it's correct because it's "always been done that way." The only way to find a better solution is to start with first principles and to work forward, which is something I finally did.

By applying the correct biomechanics and understanding the forces of movement of the spine, you can see that the pedicle screw is a suboptimal device for immobilizing the spine. This argument does not say that pedicle screws are an air ball and completely ineffective. Sometimes when the bone is healthy, a decent fixation can be achieved. However, this fixation is nowhere close to what the surgeon believes the patient is getting.

For the past two to three decades, we have tested this construct based on pullout strength. Each time we have tried to augment the screw, we focused on the pullout strength. However, it turns out that screws do not fail in pullout but in toggle. The toggle is the primary event. Once the toggle loosens the screw, then the spine falls forward because the surgery has stripped all the paraspinal muscles. In scoliosis, that is when proximal junctional kyphosis occurs. Therefore, the proximal junctional kyphosis is a direct side effect of using pedicle screws in scoliosis surgeries.

The Biomechanics of Intervertebral Graft

This book is written for the general public. Just in case a spine surgeon ends up reading this book, I want to take a moment to discuss a very important topic in the world of spine surgery that remains open to considerable debate.

In my field, the whole goal is to do whatever is in the surgeon's power to increase the chance of the fusion solidifying. As I mentioned in previous chapters, this is a very difficult thing to do. The misapplication of fracture healing to spinal fusion is an example of doctors going down the wrong road. In fracture fixation, we are talking about healing the bones. In lumbar fusion, we are trying to create bone where there was no bone before. Therefore, the biomechanics and the physiology are completely different.

Overall, there are four different ways or trajectories to place a spacer between the two vertebral bodies, such as L4 and L5. One is the anterior approach, when the surgeon goes from the front, pushing the abdominal contents to the side. This is called *ALIF*. The spine is viewed from the front, the disc is taken out, and a spacer is placed between the two vertebrae. The second way of placing a spacer between the two vertebral bodies is through the side. That is a procedure called *XLIF*. With this approach, you go through the side, dissect the psoas muscles, and insert a graft between the vertebral bodies. The third way is from the back. With this surgery, you do a laminectomy, enter the spinal canal, push the nerves to the side, and access the intervertebral space. As you have pushed the nerves to the side, you can insert the spacer between the two vertebrae. This is called *PLIF*.

The fourth method is a trajectory between the side and the back approach. We call this surgery *TLIF*.

As you can see, there are four different ways of performing the same type of surgery. In each, the surgeon is taking the cartilage of the disc between the two vertebral bodies and placing a cage that is packed with either bone substitute or bone graft, promoting fusion between the two vertebral bodies. A side anterior approach is possible but not common.

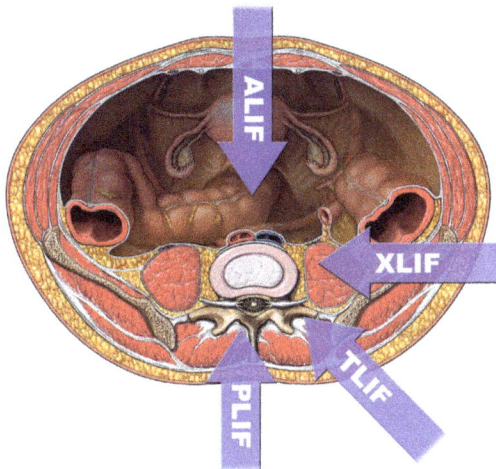

Figure 32: Lumbar Interbody Fusion Techniques

To this day, there is no solid evidence to prove which procedure is superior. Each procedure has its positives and negatives. I won't go into a lot more detail, but I want to note that the approach a surgeon uses has a lot to do with his or her training and experience. For example, an anterior approach, especially at the level of L4-5, requires the utilization of an abdominal surgeon or trauma surgeon that is very familiar with dissection or repair of the great vessels. If you do not have the availability of a great abdominal surgeon in your practice, it will limit the option for an anterior interbody fusion.

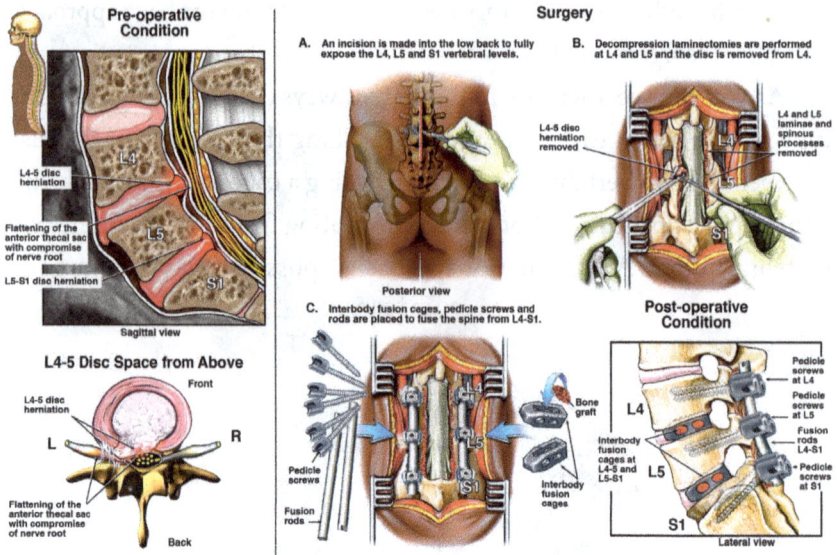

**Figure 33: L 4-5 and L5-S1 Disc Herniations
with Posterior Discectomy Fusion**

However, the interbody fusion helps the overall fusion by two means. One way is by creating a space where the fusion can take place. It helps with the surface area that is available for the bone to grow between the two vertebrae. The second way is stability, though such stability is a much-debated topic in the world of spine surgery.

Some surgeons view the disc as pretty much nonexistent in adding stability to the construct. In their view, if they do not see bone or metal, then it almost does not count. Their perception is that the spine is like a building, and you have to place a graft so that it does not fall down.

I disagree with that thought process. The disc is cartilage and is composed of water, which is not compressible. It cannot be seen on the X-ray, but it significantly contributes to the stability of the spine. If the disc was not there, the entire vertebrae would collapse completely. Therefore, the disc contributes to the overall stability of the spine.

Except when standing straight, as I discussed earlier, the spine goes through motion. That motion is flexion or rotation of vertebra relative to the vertebra below with the axis going through the middle of the disc space. Let's see how an interbody graft tries to stop this motion. In a way, when you put a graft into an intervertebral space, it is not secured to the vertebra above and below with a device. Therefore, it does not add to the rigidity of the construct of the spine that we are trying to fuse. The graft contributes to the ability of the spine to resist the flexion motion.

I watched my children play Jenga and noticed that it was exactly what I do in my work. In a normal motion segment (the vertebra above and below with the disc in between), the axis of rotation is in the middle of the disc space. By removing the disc and placing a graft, you change the axis of rotation. The best place to put the graft is as anterior as possible. It is best for the graft to stick out by 1 mm. However, that is something that surgeons do not like to do because there are always very vital structures anterior to the vertebra. The best placement of the graft is anterior enough that it is at least flush with the anterior longitudinal ligament.

Why is the best placement of the graft as anteriorly as possible? When the graft is placed anteriorly, the axis of rotation is moved anteriorly. Now, instead of the axis of rotation of L4 over L5 at the middle of the L4-5 disc space, the axis of the rotation now transfers anteriorly to the anterior and inferior lip of the L4 vertebra. This way, the vertebral column is more stable, and it takes a little bit more to displace the spine anteriorly and to destabilize it. The interbody graft contributes to stability but not by much. Its contribution is more so for the surface for fusion than for actual mechanical stability. That is one of the reasons that research so far has not been able to find a difference between the techniques of interbody fusion. In a way, whatever the surgeon is comfortable with or whatever they have available to them can be implemented, even though the anterior approach would theoretically be the most stable.

A Better Device to Immobilize
Spinal Vertebra Efficiently

The problem of finding a better device to efficiently immobilize spinal vertebrae is something I have been working on for several years and have found a theoretical solution. My solution is theoretical because no clinical studies have yet been initiated to test it. I am hopeful that my colleagues will embrace the challenge. My goal, which I originally thought was fairly modest, has grown and turned into something that I never imagined. It got so big that I had to stop work, the reasons for which I will explain at the end of this section.

Understanding the true biomechanics of the spine can easily explain why the current methods that we use are ineffective. In brief, the pedicle screw is ineffective because the forces do not distribute along the length of the screw in a uniform fashion, and there are pressure points. This makes it much easier for failure to occur in any system. Additionally, it uses the cancellous bone to immobilize the spine. Right away, the screw is at a disadvantage. Taking into account the true biomechanics of the spine, the interbody graft also contributes a small amount to the overall stability of the construct. What should be done?

When I set out to invent a device, I had two ways that I could go. One way was to improve on a device already available to us. That would be an invention that could make the screw work better. However, that route has already been exhausted over the past three decades. Everything we do to improve screw function improves it regarding pullout, but the failure happens in toggle. I knew that making a better screw was not the appropriate device. I needed to develop a completely new device to immobilize the vertebrae.

To do that, I worked backward. I first asked myself where the strongest bone in the vertebrae is. I also asked whether this strong bone is anatomically available without risks to the patient. As I explained

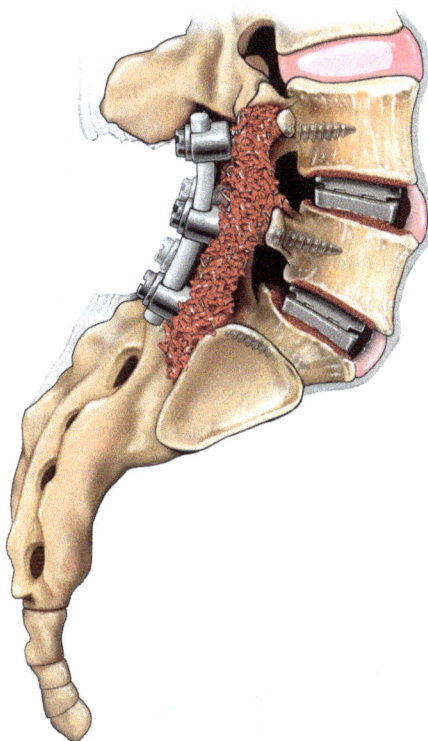

Figure 34: Spine Fusion Rods

previously, the strongest bone in the vertebrae is what we call the lamina. The lamina is the roof of the spinal canal. The lamina is one of the strongest bones in the body, and it stays very strong even in the elderly, as it does not get affected by osteoporosis. Therefore, this bone seems appropriate as an anchor point. We have used lamina for an anchor in the past, but with devices that were not appropriate, such as sublaminar wire, which is threaded under the lamina and twisted over a rod. We also used hooks. These are both inappropriate devices and did not function very well. However, they showed that the lamina could be used as a point of anchor.

The next question was how to grab and hold on to the lamina so it can be as rigid as possible. That is when I came up with the idea for the Aslie Laminar Plating System (ALPS). Lamina is a flat bone by itself, and it has two sharp edges on each side. I knew that whatever was going to hold on to the lamina would need to be able to make this sharp turn without causing pressure points and had to be able to hold both sides of a flat bone without losing grip. There is no metal that can behave this way, so this device needed to be made with a flexible material.

I initially came up with the idea to place a flat plate behind the lamina on one side to distribute the force along the entire surface of the lamina on one side. To secure this plate against the lamina, something flexible would be required with properties of being rigid as well without loosening.

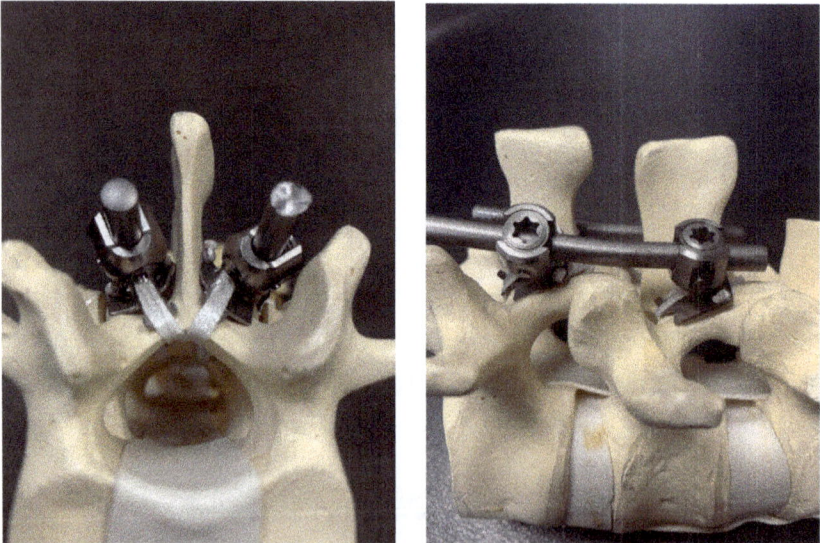

Figure 35: ALPS (Aslie Laminar Plating System)

There were six steps that we needed to overcome for the project to materialize. The first step was to see if there is an appropriate strap

222

available to us. I took different suture materials from the operating room home to test the strength. I trialed suture material after suture material, but I was getting disappointed. There was no material that would be strong enough to provide rigid fixation and hold the spine together. This material needed to be flexible, but also something that would not stretch in size over time, or fixation would be lost. It would also need enough flexibility not to cause pressure points on the bone.

Eventually, my bioengineer was able to find a material called Dyneema, which are straps made of polyethylene strands. Knee replacements and hip replacement components are made of this substance. The material is stronger than the same size steel cables and also flexible at the same time. It turned out there was only one place in the world making medical-grade Dyneema—in Switzerland. We had to order this specially made, as it had to be a specific braid and specific size to be used in our experiments.

The day my bioengineer called to say that the strap had arrived from Switzerland, I immediately flew to Santa Cruz to inspect it. I was very surprised. I brought some of the material home with me to test in my own office. Whatever I tested in my office was just to give us an idea and was unofficial. The lab that I set up and the world-class bioengineers I hired were very capable of following the regulations and knowing the FDA standards, as they had been previously involved with the development of another approved device.

The materials worked better than expected, so then the question was how to secure the strap to the plate. I knew I eventually had to use a rod for the fixation because that had worked well, especially in the world of scoliosis. We had tulips that could secure the screws into the rod. However, we had to develop a way to secure the tulip to the plate and needed to develop a clamp for the Dyneema. That is when the idea came to me that we had to build the clamp into the base of the tulip, and this material had to be titanium.

I can tell you that building this clamp was an absolute engineering marvel. This would not have been possible ten years earlier, as we had to use laser drilling because the dimensions were so small. Building a strong clamp at the base of the tulip turned out to be a very complex process. I have learned in life that everything that comes with positives also comes with negatives. The positive properties that make Dyneema very good also make it very challenging to work with. As you know, this is the same material that hip replacements and knee replacements are made of, and the strap is very slippery, so clamping it became a challenge. In addition, the material could not be crushed because it would break, and that would rip the construct. I cannot tell you how many prototypes we had to go through and how many clamps we made to come up with the shoe that would be able to clamp the Dyneema so that it would hold on to something very slippery, and at the same time, not crush it.

I had the good fortune of working with extremely smart people. However, as I was developing this device, there was something even more important that was happening: my understanding of the spine and biomechanics. During the four years I spent developing this device and the five years subsequent to that, I came to understand the biomechanics of the spine perhaps better than anyone else in the world.

The Wolverine Phenomenon

When a surgeon places screws, he always has to place them based on the angle of the pedicle. He has to follow that angle so that the screw can be inserted into the pedicle safely. That is not such an easy thing to do, because the facet joint is right on top of the pedicle where you want to insert the screw. The facet joint is like a dome. That is the reason it is very difficult to find a perfect starting position for the pedicle screw to be in the middle. The surgeon sometimes struggles in terms of fighting the muscle to angle the screw medially. Every surgeon puts the screws in freehand, usually under live X-rays. There is absolutely no way that a surgeon can put the screws in a straight line, all lined up perfectly.

Most spine surgeons are under the impression that the multiaxial tulip can compensate for the different angles of the screw heads. This is a misconception. The final resting place of the rod is defined by the screw head because that is where the rod is going to eventually sit, once the bolts are tightened. When six screws are placed on each side to fuse five levels, there is no way the screw heads can line up perfectly in a straight line, or whatever the angle of the spine is. When the screws are connected, some of the screws start fighting each other. In some cases, based on the bone quality, some of the screws can fail right off the bat.

I call this the "Wolverine phenomenon," from X-Men, because of the claws. Tightening the screws to the rod creates claws inside the vertebra that cause some of the screws to cut out of the bone by just placing the rod. I estimate in some cases, you can lose almost 40 percent of the fixation, and the patient has not even gotten to the recovery room yet. This phenomenon is a direct result of using pedicle screws.

I discovered this phenomenon because I saw a similar thing with my device. I had to go back and study the pedicle screws critically, and I found out that they were suffering from the same problem. The position of the tulip cannot be changed in relation to the screw because the screw has one shaft. However, the position of the tulip can be changed over the plate in the back of the lamina. I was able to solve that problem in my device. When the plate sits behind the lamina and it gets tightened, the tulips line up perfectly. That reduces the tension and makes the placement of the rod much easier for the surgeon. This is another potential benefit of the laminar plating system over the pedicle screw system. In this way, there is no Wolverine phenomenon because the plate is contoured. That means it can sit in only one place, which makes ALPS placement very consistent from surgeon to surgeon and from surgery to surgery. The final result is always the same in every surgery.

So far, we have talked about the lamina being the anchor point by using a flat plate against the lamina for distribution of the force and using a composite strap to hold the plate in place. The next step would be to determine if the placement is safe and whether it compromises any anatomy.

The answer is very obvious. We have used sublaminar wires with relative ease in the past. There were some problems with neurological damage using sublaminar wires, but because the straps in laminar plating are flexible, they cannot cause any injury to the neural structures.

The next step would be to come up with a plate that is contoured to the back of the lamina. Of course, the lamina is different in every region of the spine. There is the cervical spine, the thoracic spine, and the lumbar spine. That means that the plate can be contoured to the back of the lamina in separate regions.

We tested ALPS in our laboratory, and the results were astounding. An entire person could be hung from one of these devices. The strength of this device is far beyond the physiological loads that would be applied, and it has not even been optimized yet.

Reception Among Surgeons

I presented my device to the Congress of Neurological Surgeons in 2015, and I won a place in the Innovations Showcase. That meant the surgeons in charge of the Innovations Showcase found my device acceptable and worthy to be presented to the rest of the world of neurosurgery. The reception was fantastic. I showed it to different surgeons, and some of the surgeons asked if it was available to use right away. That was very good news for me, and I was very honored. However, my device was in the prototype stages and still needed to be tested inside a human being. That is when I started approaching different instrument companies. I was shocked by what I found out.

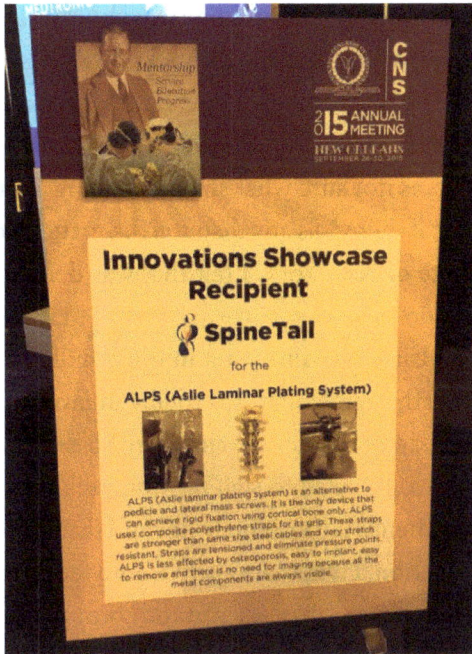

Figure 36: ALPS at the Congress of Neurological Surgeons 2015

I started out talking to representatives of four major companies to get introduced to the respective heads of development for devices. The people who were in charge of development were very excited. They asked me to make a formal presentation of the device to their companies. After talking one to two hours on the phone or in-person at conferences, at the end of the conversation, they told me that all I had to do was sign a nondisclosure agreement. I got the nondisclosure agreement and showed it to my patent lawyer. My patent lawyer stated he did not see anything unusual. I felt pretty good about this and was thinking about signing it.

My wife happens to be a very well-known trial lawyer in California. She specializes in nursing home advocacy and represents patients that are neglected in nursing homes. I approached my wife and asked her to review my nondisclosure agreement. She was shocked by what she read. One of the sentences said that "Dr. Aslie acknowledges the fact that this company can develop this device independently even after his presentation." That was nothing. My wife asked me if I wanted to go to New York many times, but I was not sure what she was talking about. She said the contract stated that if there was any dispute, the matter would need to be litigated in the State of New York. I felt that was definitely something I would not want to do.

As my wife explained the fine print in the nondisclosure agreement, it became clear that the agreement was totally in favor of the instrument company. I contacted the head of development to explain my dilemma. I advised them they would need to sign *my* nondisclosure agreement, but the head of development said absolutely not and that they have lawyers to take care of this situation. I told them there were a few parts of the nondisclosure agreement that were absolutely in the company's favor and would need to be changed. I was told that it would be impossible to make any changes and that I would need to take it or leave it. I could not believe this. I wondered if they did not want to see my presentation but just wanted to steal my idea. I wondered at that time how many surgeons had already signed those NDAs not knowing that they had lost their inventions.

In the meantime, my knowledge of spine surgery continued to increase. As I was progressing through the development and prototyping of my device, I realized that the current papers and experiments were showing that the pedicle screw does not work. This was happening at the same time. I also began to realize how instrument companies are able to impose their will on the world of spine surgery through the use of some of their consultants.

One time, I got up at a meeting of the American Academy of Orthopaedic Surgeons and raised the issue. I stated bluntly that, so far, every experiment had shown that pedicle screws do not increase fusion rate and do not improve outcome. I asked how we would address this issue.

One of the surgeons on the panel of discussion accused me of just trying to promote my own device. I tried to explain that it was the other way around. It was because I was developing this device that I studied the pedicle screw in more detail and found out that we have been using the wrong biomechanics for the treatment of spinal conditions. My discovery took place over five years of conducting experiments and questioning the literature.

That comment made a very important impact on my decision-making. When I started my research and development, my goal was monetary. I wanted to create a device that would become successful and bring me financial benefit. As my device and my experimentation deepened, I realized the problem we are facing in spine surgery is not just biology and not just the aging population. The problem I discovered was much bigger than I thought.

I never considered that I would stumble onto such a huge problem and spend five years looking for the answers. From the inception of spine surgery, we have chosen the wrong path. We have done everything in spine surgery based on what we learned in general orthopedics. As I have mentioned previously, this is wrong. The spine is a much more complex entity, and we should have never applied what we learned in general orthopedics to spine surgery.

The fact I am stating is not popular among surgeons. Based on my research and analysis, I believe that spine surgery was never meant to be a subspecialty of orthopedic surgery or neurosurgery. Spine surgery should be treated as a specialty by itself, and I believe the very least we can do is to increase the exposure to spine surgery in these subspecialties, especially in orthopedic surgery.

Once I found out the magnitude of the problem, things changed for me. We are talking about an entire specialty for the entirety of humanity. This is a much bigger issue than one person, and it potentially affects every person on this planet. I had to stop the development of my device just to make sure that my message does not get lost in the bigger picture. I wanted to make sure there would be no accusation of my injecting my own bias into the discussion. I realized that I could not criticize an instrument company for injecting their bias if I could be accused of promoting my own bias on the other end. I am willing to sacrifice myself and my future to get this message out. At this time, it is not about me getting a vacation home or driving a nice car. It is about the entire population with back issues getting proper care. It is much bigger than one person. That is the reason I stopped developing my device. I truly believe that the entire practice of spine surgery needs an attitude adjustment. Who says that instrumentation must fail? What about instrumentation that lasts you a lifetime? How about instrumentation that doesn't rely on fusion? I promise you I will deliver that in my lifetime.

I have even bigger goals now than what I have already stated. Spine surgery is a very technical surgery, and a significant amount of equipment is required. When the screws are placed, a neuromonitoring technician must be in the room, and imaging is required in the form of X-rays with its technician. This makes spine surgery with the use of pedicle screws extremely expensive. There are many hospitals throughout the world that do not have access to this type of equipment. When the pedicle screw is inserted into a patient, an imaging study is needed to make sure the screw does not penetrate important structures and create significant morbidity. The laminar plating system that I developed uses composite straps, and imaging would not be required to pass it under the lamina. It is a very flexible device, and the part in the canal is not going to cause any neurological damage. In addition, there is no need for imaging studies because the metal part of the device is all visible to the surgeon.

Right now, the attitude in the world of spine surgery is that instrumentation, in the form of adding screws, is a temporary scaffolding for the fusion that is to take place. Every spine surgeon knows and tells you when we put those screws in there, it's a race between fusion taking place and screws failing.

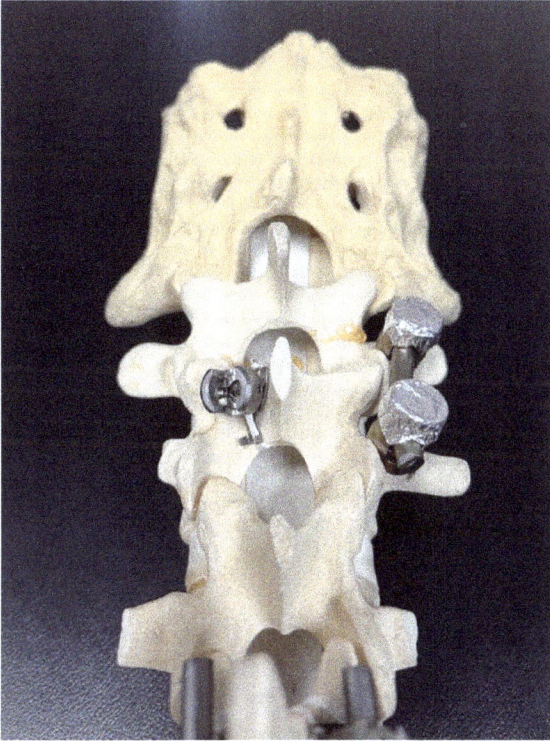

Figure 37: Screws Attached to the Vertebrae (Laminar plating system and pedicle screw system side by side. ALPS is much more medial than pedicle screws and therefore requires much less dissection.)

With the Aslie Laminar Plating System, in the future we can have instrumentation that does not rely on fusion but can give close to a 100 percent fusion rate if desired. With pedicle screws, there is no room for improvement. The screw is what you get. With the ALPS system, we can modify the strap or plate to give us optimized function.

Every time I do a fusion surgery, my room is full of equipment. The screw system needs at least six to eight large trays. Screws come in all lengths and diameters. ALPS, on the other hand, will come in a standardized shape. There are cervical, thoracic, and lumbar types. That means the surgeon will need only one tray of equipment. There would be no need for X-rays or neuromonitoring either. Therefore, even less well-equipped rural communities will have access to spine surgery.

If my device is approved for use, spine surgery could become available in developing countries; developed countries would not be the only place that has access to spinal surgery. My ultimate goal now is to make spine surgery simple enough and successful enough to be available to anyone who needs it, even in the most rural communities. I firmly expect that will be my contribution to the world of medicine and civilization.

Sources Cited

Abdu, William A., Olivia A. Sacks, Anna N.A. Tosteson, Wenyan Zhao, Tor D. Tosteson, Tamara S. Morgan, Adam Pearson, James N. Weinstein, and Jon D. Lurie. 2018. "Long-Term Results of Surgery Compared with Nonoperative Treatment for Lumbar Degenerative Spondylolisthesis in the Spine Patient Outcomes Research Trial (SPORT)." *Spine* 43 (23): 1619-30. doi: 10.1097/BRS.0000000000002682

Abelson, Reed. 2006. "Whistle-Blower Suit Says Device Maker Generously Rewards Doctors." *New York Times*, January 24, 2006. https://www.nytimes.com/2006/01/24/business/whistleblower-suit-says-device-maker-generously-rewards-doctors.html

BMTN Staff. 2018. "Senate Panel Says Medtronic Edited Clinical Studies to Tout Spine Product." *Bring Me The News*, March 8, 2018. https://bringmethenews.com/news/senate-panel-says-medtronic-manipulated-articles-to-tout-spine-products

Carragee, Eugene J., Alexander J. Ghanayem, Bradley K. Weiner, David J. Rothman, and Christopher M. Bono. 2011. "A Challenge to Integrity in Spine Publications: Years of Living Dangerously with the Promotion of Bone Growth Factors." *The Spine Journal*, 11 (6), 463-8. https://www.thespinejournalonline.com/article/S1529-9430(11)00353-6/fulltext#%20.DOI:https://doi.org/10.1016/j.spinee.2011.06.001

Carreyrou, John, and Tom McGinty. 2011. "Medtronic Surgeons Held Back, Study Says." *Wall Street Journal*, June 29, 2011. https://www.wsj.com/articles/SB10001424052702303627104576413663395567784

Chris Wilcox vs. Medtronic Inc. et al. US District Court Eastern District of Louisiana. 2013. https://aboutlawsuits-wpengine.netdna-ssl.com/wp-content/uploads/2013-06-06-Wilcox-Complaint.pdf

Daniel Fanning et al. and Margaret Schmerling et al. v. AcroMed Corporation. US District Court for the Eastern District of Pennsylvania. 1997. https://www.paed.uscourts.gov/documents/opinions/97D1164P.pdf

Eisner, Walter. 2017. "FDA Reclassifies Pedicle Screws." *Orthopedics This Week*, January 24, 2017. https://ryortho.com/breaking/fda-reclassifies-pedicle-screws/

Fauber, John. 2012. "The $34-Million Spine Surgeon." *Milwaukee Journal Sentinel/MedPage Today*, October 25, 2012. https://www.medpagetoday.com/painmanagement/backpain/35550

Fauber, John. 2014. "Medtronic to pay $22 million to settle legal claims over spine product." *Milwaukee Journal Sentinel*, May 6, 2014. https://archive.jsonline.com/watchdog/watchdogreports/medtronic-to-pay-22-million-to-settle-legal-claims-over-spine-product-b99263776z1-258155261.html/

Meier, Barry. 2013. "Outside Review of Clinical Data Finds a Spinal Treatment's Benefit Overstated." *New York Times*, June 17, 2013. https://www.nytimes.com/2013/06/18/business/infuse-a-spinal-treatment-found-no-better-than-older-remedy.html

Moore, Janet. 2009. "Lawsuit Against Surgeons Dismissed." *StarTribune*, March 20, 2009. https://www.startribune.com/lawsuit-against-surgeons-dismissed/41609942/

NASSspine. "Dr. Carragee of *The Spine Journal*, Discusses InFuse, Medtronic and Scientific Publishing on *CNN*." YouTube video, 4:25, November 1, 2012. https://www.youtube.com/watch?v=kfa4_M5FKfo

Staff of the Committee on Finance. 2012. "Staff Report on Medtronic's Influence on Infuse Clinical Studies. US Senate." October 2012. https://www.finance.senate.gov/imo/media/doc/Medtronic_Report3.pdf

Steigenga, Jennifer T., Khalaf F. al-Shammari, Francisco H. Nociti, Carl E. Misch, and Hom-Lay Wang. 2003. "Dental Implant Design and Its Relationship to Long-Term Implant Success." *Implant Dentistry*, 12 (4): 306-17. doi: 10.1097/01.id.0000091140.76130.a1

Thomsen, Karsten, Finn B. Christensen, Søren P. Eiskjær, Ebbe S. Hansen, Søren Fruensgaard, and Cody E. Bünger. 1997. "1997 Volvo Award Winner in Clinical Studies. The Effect of Pedicle Screw Instrumentation on Functional Outcome and Fusion Rates in Posterolateral Lumbar Spinal Fusion: A Prospective, Randomized Clinical Study." *Spine*, 22 (24): 2813-22. https://doi. org/10.1097/00007632-199712150-00004

Times Staff and Wire Reports. 1996. "Medical Firm AcroMed Agrees to Settle Suit." *Los Angeles Times*, December 9, 1996. https://www.latimes.com/ archives/la-xpm-1996-12-09-fi-7389-story.html

Weiser, Benjamin, and John Schwartz. 1996. "The Tangled Path of FDA Review." *Washington Post*, March 29, 1996. https://www.washingtonpost.com/ archive/politics/1996/03/29/the-tangled-path-of-fda-review/3e7fe546-8f31-415e-89d6-788686a1285e/

Zdeblick, Thomas A. (1993). "A Prospective, Randomized Study of Lumbar Fusion. Preliminary Results." *Spine*, 18 (8): 983-91. https://doi.org/ 10.1097/00007632-199306150-00006

Index

Note: Page numbers in *italics* indicate photographs and illustrations.